PENGUIN CLASSICS

MERITS OF THE PLAGUE

IBN HAJAR AL-ASQALANI (d. 852/1449) was a master of prophetic traditions, a prodigious historian and biographer, a chief judge on the highest court in the Mamluk Sultanate, and a trader raised by a powerful family of spice merchants. His world was shaped by the legacy of the Black Death; indeed, he lost three of his children to the plague. His masterpiece was a multivolume commentary on prophetic traditions called *Fatḥ al-Bārī* (The Divine Aid to Victory), parts of which he incorporated into *Merits of the Plague*. He authored religious poetry and several voluminous histories and biographical dictionaries that chronicled events and notable persons of the seventh and eighth Islamic centuries. His works are still consulted today by historians and religious scholars alike.

JOEL BLECHER is Associate Professor of History at The George Washington University and the author of *Said the Prophet of God: Hadith Commentary across a Millennium*, which has been translated into Arabic. He is the author of numerous articles, and his work has been supported by the National Endowment for the Humanities, the American Council of Learned Societies, the Institute for Advanced Study at Princeton, and the Kluge Center at the Library of Congress. He has spoken about the Islamic world on public radio and numerous podcasts, and has contributed to *The Atlantic*.

MAIRAJ SYED is Associate Professor of Religious Studies, Middle East and South Asia Studies, and former director of the Medieval and Early Modern Studies program at the University of California, Davis. He is the author of *Coercion and Responsibility in Islam: A Study in Ethics and Law*, and many articles on Islamic thought. He is the recipient of numerous awards and grants for his research, including a Fulbright Fellowship.

IBN HAJAR
AL-ASQALANI

Merits of the Plague

Edited, Translated, and with
an Introduction and Notes by
JOEL BLECHER *and* MAIRAJ SYED

PENGUIN BOOKS

PENGUIN BOOKS

An imprint of Penguin Random House LLC
penguinrandomhouse.com

Map design by Joel Blecher and Mairaj Syed
Map cartography by Bill Nelson

LIBRARY OF CONGRESS CATALOGING-IN-PUBLICATION DATA
Names: Ibn Ḥajar al-ʿAsqalānī, Aḥmad ibn ʿAlī, 1372–1449 author. |
Blecher, Joel, 1982- editor, translator. | Syed, Mairaj U., editor, translator.
Title: Merits of the plague / Ibn Hajar al-ʿAsqalānī ; edited, translated,
and with an Introduction and Notes by Joel Blecher, and Mairaj Syed.
Includes bibliographical references and index.
Identifiers: LCCN 2022037454 (print) | LCCN 2022037455 (ebook) |
ISBN 9780143136613 (paperback) | ISBN 9780525508113 (ebook)
Subjects: LCSH: Plague—Religious aspects—Islam. | Plague—History—Early works to 1800.
Classification: LCC RC172 .I26 2023 (print) | LCC RC172 (ebook) |
DDC 614.5/732—dc23/eng/20221011
LC record available at https://lccn.loc.gov/2022037454
LC ebook record available at https://lccn.loc.gov/2022037455

Printed in the United States of America
2nd Printing

Set in Sabon LT Pro

For Aria and Hawthorn

For Taj and Zakira Syed

and

For those lost in the pandemic

Contents

Introduction by JOEL BLECHER *and* MAIRAJ SYED ix
Suggestions for Further Reading xxxvii
A Note on the Translation xli
Chronology li
Maps lvi

MERITS OF THE PLAGUE

Preface of the Author 1
CHAPTER ONE
Origins of the Plague 3
CHAPTER TWO
Understanding the Plague 13
CHAPTER THREE
Martyrdom and the Plague 67
CHAPTER FOUR
Against Flight from the Plague 95
CHAPTER FIVE
When the Plague Strikes 155
EPILOGUE
A Record of Plagues 189

Appendix: From Ibn Ḥajar's "Journal of the Plague Years" 219
Glossary and Register of Proper Names 227
Notes 233
Index 255

Introduction

This book was conceived in the spring of 2020, during the early days of the coronavirus pandemic as dread, chaos, lockdowns, and death gripped the world. Struggling to absorb our new circumstances, many readers, ourselves included, turned to classic works on the plague with fresh eyes. Those works offered a sort of brutal comfort, a reminder that humans have faced times like these in the past—indeed, times much worse than these—and made sense of them. Passages crafted hundreds of years ago or more, which once seemed arcane and fanciful, now offered profound insights across time and spoke to our current moment of astonishment and despair. Reports of the plague's daily death tolls that scholars once viewed as inaccurately high now seemed comically low.

In relative terms, the deadliest pandemic in human history was surely the Black Death, which began in the thirteenth century, peaked in the fourteenth century, and recurred periodically for more than four centuries afterward.[1] Even though many modern readers will associate the Black Death primarily as a moment in medieval European history—and plague literature from the Western canon has returned to our bookshelves and nightstands with a vengeance—some of the most profound meditations on the plague were arguably produced outside the West, in the lingua franca of Arabic, and in the cultural and intellectual milieu of Islam. Perhaps this is because Muslim writers, whose audiences crisscrossed Africa and Eurasia for trade, study, and pilgrimage, were best positioned to grasp the truly global scope of the plague and the moral, theological, political, and economic dilemmas it posed.

One of the most important and influential works on the plague in Islamic thought is Ibn Ḥajar al-ʿAsqalānī's *Merits of the Plague*, a fifteenth-century book that is here translated from Arabic to English for the first time. The book wrestles with debates over the origins of the disease, the most effective responses to it, and the meaning of suffering and mass death. In doing so, the author crafts a compelling, if counterintuitive, argument: there is merit in the plague if one understands it as an expression of God's will and an opportunity to practice patience and care for others. To make this case, the author weaves together evidence from stories about the Prophet Muhammad and his Companions, medical works, law books, anecdotes from firsthand experiences, tales of unseen spirits, death-count registers, and plague-era poetry that spans eight centuries and the known Muslim world. In this way, *Merits of the Plague* is both a profound meditation on the plague as well as a classical anthology of medicine, law, history, traditions, and literature about pandemics in the pre-modern world.

Ibn Ḥajar al-ʿAsqalānī, a fifteenth-century Egyptian, a paragon of the Islamic intellectual tradition, was at one time the most powerful judge in the Mamluk Empire. He was also a poet, a merchant, and a once-in-a-generation scholar whose knowledge of the Hadith (the corpus of narratives involving the Prophet Muhammad) was renowned from North Africa to India. The fact that he was stricken by the disease, and lost three children to it, must have had a profound effect on his thinking. He wrote this short volume to serve an audience coming to terms with the new realities brought about by the plague: widespread death, uncertainty, fear of contagion, the limitations of medicine, and crises of faith. While these themes will ring familiar to all readers who lived through the recent pandemic, the book also invites us into a world and a vision of reality inflected by Islamic thought, where the jinn meddle in human affairs and the heavenly rewards of martyrdom give meaning to suffering and the great loss of life.

After Ibn Ḥajar's death, *Merits of the Plague* was abridged and adapted by his students for new audiences, and continued to be read throughout the Ottoman period in the centuries that followed. Just as readers in our own day have turned to *The Decameron* of Boccaccio, *The Betrothed* of Manzoni, and Defoe's *A Journal of the Plague Year*, Ibn Ḥajar's book has also garnered renewed interest in the wake of the coronavirus among Muslims, as well as among scholars and public intellectuals interested in historical responses to pandemics outside Europe, for which few accessible translations on the subject exist. Readers opening up the *New York Times*'s opinion page in the spring of 2020 would have been greeted by the invocation of Ibn Ḥajar's work on the plague in the service of imploring the Saudi government to suspend the hajj.[2]

Indeed, it is a sad but telling irony that the most influential book on the plague in our own era, Camus's *La Peste*—which is set in a modern Algerian port city that had been controlled by Muslims during the era of the Black Death—fails to include a single Muslim character, much less any mention of this or any other treasury of Islamic knowledge on the plague, works that must have been circulating in the city's libraries and studied in homes, seminaries, and places of worship for centuries. Perhaps this glaring omission underlines Camus's own critique of the alienation produced by modern life, as people are increasingly divided from one another and from their own rich histories. We hope this translation will serve as one small step in repairing those divisions and broken links.

I. PLAGUE AND EPIDEMICS IN ISLAMIC HISTORY

Was Islam formed, in a sense, by the plague? Although the Qur'an makes no explicit mention of the plague as such, historical sources suggest that it was. We know, for instance, that the Plague of Justinian, which began in 541, cyclically reoccurred during the early Islamic incursions into Byzantium and in the era of the Umayyad Caliphate (661–750). Indeed, as some scholars have argued, the devastation of the plague may have been an important factor in weakening the Byzantine Empire, helping, alongside other political and economic factors, to open a space for the ascendance of Islam outside of Arabia. The Umayyads, who displaced the Byzantine Empire in Greater Syria, likewise may have seen its leaders and its population decimated by later outbreaks of this plague, opening a space for the Abbasid revolution in the year 750.[3]

This is to say nothing of the Prophet Muhammad's narratives, or hadiths, that circulated and were collected during this early period, which depict the Prophet as guiding his community amid the spread of infectious diseases and the foretelling of plagues to come. While the Prophet himself was not known to have experienced the plague, the hadiths portray the first caliphs as confronting it in Syria and turning for guidance to the Prophet's hadith on contagion and his prophecies of the coming plague. Plague during these eras thus provoked intense interest not only among Muslim audiences learned in Greek medical literature, but also among those early Muslim jurists and theologians who struggled to make sense of what message God might have intended to send in delivering a plague to seemingly innocent Muslims. Was it a punishment? If so, for what reason? Was it an opportunity for heavenly reward? If so, how?

Devastating as these early and successive waves of plague were, the Black Death that peaked in the mid-fourteenth century stands out for its geographical reach and the sheer magnitude of the death toll. If we consider the natural history of that plague—the spread of the bacterium *Yersinia pestis*—there is no shortage of possible vectors. While several locales of geographic origination have been hypothesized, the Tibetan Plateau is most commonly cited, with Crimea serving as the proximate hot spot by which the plague entered the Mediterranean littoral. Some scholars have argued that the plague may have been spread by the natural migration of flea-borne rodents, camels, and other animals, but human migrations—for trade, pilgrimage, and war—must have played an important role as well. As Monica Green has recently argued, the western military expansion of the Mongols across the Tibetan Plateau and the Silk Road trading routes into the lands of Islam in the middle of the thirteenth century—in particular, "grain shipments that the Mongols brought with them to several sieges," including the 1258 siege of Baghdad—"were the most likely mechanism of transmission."[4] On this view, the outbreak in Crimea in 1346 represented a local "spillover event" from the plague reservoirs seeded by those thirteenth-century Mongol campaigns. Muslim pilgrims then brought the plague to Mecca's doorstep in 1349, when dizzying numbers of pilgrims were said to have perished.[5]

During the thirteenth to the early sixteenth centuries, Egypt, Syria, and the western province of Arabia that was home to Mecca and Medina were controlled by the Mamluk Sultanate, whose political and religious elite were based in Cairo. The Black Death and the successive outbreaks of the plague during this period not only posed a threat to life in the Mamluk Sultanate but also upended the economy at local and global scales. The plague drove up the price of wheat which was already exorbitantly high due to periods of famine and inflation. The price of goods that were perceived as having medicinal value, such as citron, quince, and pre-prepared medicinal syrups containing processed sugar and rosewater, skyrocketed. Urban depopulation grievously injured the cloth and textile industry, which was the lifeblood of Alexandria. This, in turn, harmed both the merchant class and indirectly the sultanate, which relied on the fees and taxes on such merchandise, given the sultanate's strategic position along the Red Sea trade route that linked the Mediterranean to the Indian Ocean. Meanwhile, the plague brought ruin to Egypt's irrigation system, and the depopulation in rural Egypt impoverished the very landed estates that provided the tax revenue to support the sultanate's army.[6]

The result was a kind of death spiral in which Muslim political authorities adopted yet higher regimes of urban and rural taxation, which led to more deleterious effects on the region's prosperity. Indeed, the very things that the learned class suggested to Sultan Ashraf Barsbay as the cause of the "The Great Extinction" of 1430—the extortionate rates of taxation placed upon the spice traders and other corrupt political reforms adopted by his predecessors—were also likely the consequence of decades of depopulation and economic instability caused by earlier waves of the disease.[7] The political authorities were thus destabilized by the plague through the deaths of their officers, worsening economic conditions, and crises of morality and religious legitimacy. In response, as Ibn Ḥajar's chronicle of the plague attests, the government would learn to develop new technologies of surveillance, forge new links with the religious elite, adopt stricter regulations of public space in the hopes of reining in corruption, temporarily loosen regulations over burial practices, and attempt to monopolize commerce and industries in the search for new streams of revenue.[8]

In several plagues, including at least two witnessed by Ibn Ḥajar, the government identified fornication as a cause of the moral corruption that led to the plague, and banned women, with few exceptions, from public spaces, on threat of drowning or other severe punishments.[9] Although women's voices are absent in our sources, it is clear that these restrictions caused tremendous suffering in their own right, as mothers were forbidden from entering the marketplaces. While in northern Europe religious minorities—in particular, Jews—were scapegoated in response to the Black Death, in Mamluk Cairo, by contrast, we find numerous accounts of Muslims, Christians, and Jews marching together in processionals while crying out in prayer in hopes of lifting the plague.[10] Instead, the women of Cairo and the threat they were perceived to pose to the sexual order prompted calls by some in the religious and political elite to police their movements.

As we will see in *Merits of the Plague*, more common religious responses to the plague included fasting, special prayers to God, reciting specific verses from the Qur'an or supplications in the Hadith to repel jinn—which many believed were responsible for spreading the plague—and the practice of patience and contemplation at home. Such techniques coexisted, sometimes uneasily, alongside practices familiar to the occult sciences, such as the wearing of sapphires, rubies, and talismans, and the enunciating of specific incantations to repel demons. They also complemented the practices of Greek medicine, which included bloodletting, the burning of aromatics such as camphor and sandalwood, and the eating of onions, sardines, vinegar, and citrus, which were believed by physicians trained in the Galenic tradition to counteract the corruption brought about by the plague and bring balance back to the body's humors.[11]

One area of intense debate during this period—which *Merits* crystalizes—was the cause of the disease and its transmission. The competing theories led to strong disagreements over whether people ought to be advised to stay put or flee when a plague strikes, or whether one should avoid entering places where plague was widespread. While some thinkers like Ibn Ḥajar rejected the idea of contagion, favoring theories they thought aligned better with the religious sources as well as empirical observation, numerous other scholars affirmed the notion of contagion, fueling a robust debate.[12]

In the modern period, Islam once again played an important role in the history of pandemics and infectious diseases, as the new technology of steamships allowed the hajj to become a primary vector by which cholera was transmitted from India during the colonial period. The British cited this concomitance as a reason for ramping up surveillance of the pilgrimage to Mecca, fearing it was a conduit for what they called the "twin plagues" of fundamentalism and disease.[13] In this way, both quarantines and the regulation of public health along the hajj became a theater in which colonial powers competed to advance their imperial aims. This phenomenon should be considered as a part of a larger pattern that Nükhet Varlik has recently identified as a form of "epidemiological orientalism," in which nineteenth-century Europeans constructed "the Orient . . . as a site of sickness" in their writings, discourses, and imaginations.[14] In the end, the international efforts undertaken by colonial powers to curb cholera along the hajj—however politically and commercially self-interested those efforts may have been—established a model upon which the World Health Organization would later be founded in 1948.

More recently, the Muslim religious response to COVID-19 has been substantial. Authorities in Muslim-majority countries closed mosque services during the height of the pandemic, and even changed the way they performed prayer in order to social distance. The annual pilgrimage to Mecca was canceled in

2020, as was the pilgrimage to al-Ḥusayn's mausoleum in Karbala. When mosques and pilgrimage destinations reopened, they did so with important modifications: Authorities limited attendance, and religious scholars, normally reluctant to change the structure of ritual, mandated social distancing even during the performance of congregational prayer.[15] Vaccination was mandated for those in Saudi Arabia intending to perform the hajj. Remarkably, many congregations accepted the alterations without protest.

II. IBN ḤAJAR: HIS LIFE, CAREER, AND WORLD

While less well known in the West than in the Middle East, Ibn Ḥajar al-ʿAsqalānī (d. 1449) can rightly be considered among the pantheon of Muslim luminaries that includes Avicenna (d. 1037), al-Ghazālī (d. 1111), Averroes (d. 1198), Ibn Taymiyya (d. 1328), Ibn Khaldūn (d. 1406), and Mullā Ṣadrā (d. ca. 1636). One can find Ibn Ḥajar's books proudly displayed for sale in virtually any bookstore where Islamic books are sold and in virtually every library that acquires books in Arabic. His authority is often invoked by a range of religious figures, from state-appointed muftis to mainstream TV clerics on Al Jazeera to ISIS propagandists in their e-magazines. His life was even made the subject of dramatization by an Egyptian soap opera.

In his own lifetime, Ibn Ḥajar wore many hats. He was a masterful and innovative commentator and critic of hadiths, a prodigious historian and biographer, a judge on the highest court in Mamluk Cairo, and a textile trader raised by a powerful family of spice merchants. His masterpiece is a twelve-volume commentary on hadiths called *Fatḥ al-Bārī* (The Divine Aid to Victory), excerpts of which he incorporated into *Merits of the Plague*. These works are still consulted today by modern historians and religious scholars alike.

Ibn Ḥajar was born in Cairo in 1372, some twenty-three years after the Black Death had peaked. While he was not alive to witness it, the world he inhabited had been transformed in its wake. His mother, Tujjār al-Ziftāwī, died soon after his birth, likely within a year. Although we know she came from an important family of spice traders—Kārimī merchants—Ibn Ḥajar had little memory of her, and apparently his care was informally undertaken by his older sister—his "mother after his mother"—even though she was no more than three or four years his elder. Ibn Ḥajar was fully orphaned at the age of three after his father, also a successful merchant and a judge of minor note, died of an unnamed illness. It was at this point that Ibn Ḥajar, at the direction of his father's will, was raised by one of Egypt's most powerful and wealthy spice merchants, Zakī al-Dīn al-Kharrūbī.[16]

To describe Ibn Ḥajar's guardian as powerful may be an understatement—Zakī al-Dīn was granted the title of "leader" or "chief" of the sultan's merchants, a position of great prestige, celebrity, and influence. Zakī al-Dīn not only introduced Ibn Ḥajar into the world of business and long-distance trade, but also opened up a possible path for his achievements as a scholar and religious thinker. At the age of eleven, Ibn Ḥajar accompanied al-Kharrūbī to Mecca for business and pilgrimage, and he studied the Hadith for the first time in his guardian's apartment, which had quite a view: Ibn Ḥajar remembered that he could look upon the black stone of the Kaʿba from its window.[17]

When Ibn Ḥajar was thirteen, two years after this momentous journey, which he memorialized in detail in his autobiography, al-Kharrūbī passed away, leaving Ibn Ḥajar orphaned a third time. It is at this point that Ibn al-Qattān, a man of learning from Alexandria, entered Ibn Ḥajar's life. Ibn al-Qattān is credited with mentoring Ibn Ḥajar in historical literature, as well as introducing him to some of the notable scholars of the time, with whom he would undertake intensive study over the following two decades. During this time, Ibn Ḥajar heard and collected hadiths from hundreds of transmitters as he traveled across Syria, Yemen, and the Ḥijaz in search of knowledge and trade—in Damascus alone, he reports he heard what amounted to "one thousand fascicles filled with hadiths"[18]—but he ultimately attached himself closely to a number of Egyptian hadith masters of his parents' and grandparents' generation: Zayn al-Dīn al-ʿIrāqī, Ibn al-Mulaqqin, and Abū Ḥafs al-Bulqīnī, among others.

At the age of twenty-four, Ibn Ḥajar married Uns ʿAbd al-Karīm ibn Aḥmad, a woman politically connected to the Mamluk Sultanate through her father, who served as the inspector of the army. She was a woman of high standing, and Ibn Ḥajar composed a remarkable love poem for her in the Arabic *ghazal* form during his travels abroad. Their first child, a daughter, Zayn Khātūn, was born almost four years later. Ibn Ḥajar had her tutored in reading and writing, and made sure that she too heard hadiths from the same luminaries with whom he had studied.

At the age of thirty-four, Ibn Ḥajar himself began lecturing on hadith literature at the Shaykhūniyya and several other important colleges in Cairo. It was through these lectures during the 1410s that he began working on the introduction to his magnum opus, *Fatḥ al-Bārī* (The Divine Aid to Victory), a commentary on al-Bukhārī's collection of authenticated hadiths that would take him nearly three decades to complete. Some of the hadiths in this collection discuss matters related to the plague, martyrdom, and the jinn, a subtle understanding of which would later become critical to the central themes of *Merits of the Plague*.

After receiving these teaching appointments, Ibn Ḥajar's talent became clear, and he was quickly promoted to several other administrative and legal positions, including mufti at the Palace of Justice and dean of academic and administrative affairs of Baybarsiyya college in Cairo. He also became close during this time with Sultan al-Muʾayyad Shaykh (r. 1412–1421); he was brought into the sultan's inner circle as one of his closest religious advisers and may have played a role in deepening the sultan's own religiosity. But it would not be until the reigns of Sultan Ashraf Barsbāy (r. 1422–1438) and Sultan Jaqmāq (r. 1438–1453) that Ibn Ḥajar would be appointed to the highest court as the Shāfiʿī chief judge of Egypt and Syria, a position he would hold intermittently for the rest of his life, removed and reinstated at the whim of the sultan. It was also during the reigns of Barsbāy and Jaqmāq that Ibn Ḥajar took over the librarianship of the Maḥmūdiyya, which contained thousands of manuscripts that Ibn Ḥajar cataloged over the course of his life.

Ibn Ḥajar's wife, Uns, had borne him daughters, but no son. In a fascinating incident that is illustrative of the dynamics of elite Mamluk-era marriages, Ibn Ḥajar secretly arranged to purchase his wife's domestic slave of Mongol origins named Khaṣṣ Turk and to take her as a concubine in the hope that she would bear him a son. Indeed, Ibn Ḥajar's only son, Muḥammad, was born to Khaṣṣ Turk in 1412, without Uns's knowledge. When Uns finally discovered what had transpired, she confronted her husband in an episode in which she cursed the child by suggesting he would never become a great scholar, as Ibn Ḥajar had hoped. Uns would not allow her husband to keep Khaṣṣ Turk and their son in Uns's home, where their family had been living, so Ibn Ḥajar had Khaṣṣ Turk and their son set up in another residence in Cairo.[19]

In the spring of 1416, a severe outbreak of the plague struck Cairo, and two of Ibn Ḥajar's daughters died: Ghāliya, who was eleven years old, and Fāṭima, who was just a toddler. Ibn Ḥajar cites the death toll that was registered by the government in Cairo to have reached five hundred a day, but he suspected that if one added to it the number of deaths that went unreported, it must have been higher. In the wake of losing two of his daughters and witnessing the mass death in his midst, Ibn Ḥajar apparently began to compose a book on the plague, but he was left unsatisfied with it. It would be another two decades until he completely revised it into the work translated here as *Merits of the Plague*.

The completion of *Merits of the Plague* followed the 1430 plague, which was worse, by all accounts, than the one that struck in 1416—the worst, perhaps, since the Black Death of 1347 nearly a century earlier. A contemporary of Ibn Ḥajar, the historian Ibn Taghrībirdī, called it "The Great Extinction," while another, al-Maqrīzī, called it "The Year of Evils." In Ibn Ḥajar's description of the scene that year, he writes:

> The death struck to the south in al-Qarāfa, until around three thousand had died. Those who carried the dead, washed them, and prepared graves became so scarce that they dug one large pit and cast the corpses into it. Many death shrouds were stolen. Stray dogs dug up bodies and ate the corpses' limbs. The caskets arrived in such numbers that I saw them lined up all the way from the al-Mu'minā prayer hall to the al-Qarāfa gate. They were like white vultures circling carrion. In the streets, it was as if the parade of caskets were a long string of camels tied by the tail, one following the other.[20]

It was in this year that Ibn Ḥajar's learned adult daughter and first-born, Zayn Khātūn, died of the disease while she was pregnant, and thus, in Ibn Ḥajar's view, the plague brought her "two martyrdoms."[21] Indeed, while he does not mention her death explicitly in *Merits of the Plague*, it is nearly impossible to read the passages that Ibn Ḥajar dedicates to the status of those women killed by plague while pregnant without considering his reckoning with this loss firsthand.

After the darkness of 1430, new opportunities for love and achievement came Ibn Ḥajar's way. In 1433, he took as his second wife Layla bint Maḥmūd ibn Tughān, a woman he had met during his travels in Syria. He was enamored with her and, as he had done before with Uns, waxed poetically about her in his *ghazals*—"I cure myself during the day" by studying hadiths, he wrote, "but at night I long for Layla."[22] Meanwhile, in 1439, Ibn Ḥajar at last celebrated the completion of *The Divine Aid to Victory*. If the rich feast, costing five hundred gold dinars, that accompanied the celebration is any indication, the book's completion was highly anticipated, and portions of the work had already been commissioned and delivered to potentates from Persia and North Africa, who offered him large sums in exchange for an early version.[23]

The final years of Ibn Ḥajar's life were again marked by plague. In the spring of 1444, as plague struck Egypt, Ibn Ḥajar himself noticed something under his arm:

> On Sunday night, the 5th of Ṣafar [May 24], I discovered a pain under my right armpit and a prickly source of discomfort, but went to sleep despite it. The next day, the pain increased slightly. So I went back to sleep in acceptance and full recognition that the affliction remained unchanged. By the 10th, it appeared under my armpit like a soft plum. After that, it lightened little by little until only a final portion of it remained.[24]

Such a mundane description of his struggle with a disease that killed so many of his countrymen, three of his daughters, his unborn grandchild, and dependents of his household should be understood less as a depiction of what must have been a harrowing bout with a deadly illness, and more as an exemplification of the principal argument of *Merits of the Plague*: that one should face the disease with acceptance and patience. That he overcame this disease at the age of seventy-two must have been particularly inspiring for his numerous students and followers, and Ibn Ḥajar's survival must have been taken as proof of his righteousness and high standing with God.

Ibn Ḥajar died after battling an unknown illness in 1449, just shy of a week before his seventy-seventh birthday. But plague had once again struck Cairo, and Ibn Ḥajar's passing occurred amid yet another wave of suffering and mass death from this disease.

III. THE WORK AND ITS RECEPTION

We have suggested here, as others before us have speculated, that the death of Ibn Ḥajar's daughters and the devastation of the 1430 plague that he witnessed firsthand must have inspired him, at least in part, to write this book. However, Ibn Ḥajar himself pointed to two motivations: one that prompted him to start it, in 1416, and the other that inspired him to finish it, in 1429. On the former, he noted in the preface that he started writing the book in response to his colleagues' request that he "collect all reports on the plague, comment on the anomalous ones, facilitate an understanding of them, interpret them, clarify their implications for the religious law, and give an account of their types."[25] On the latter, he pointed to his involvement in what he thought was a corrupt religious practice related to the plague. He observed that the people, led by the ruling elite and religious authorities, would gather in the desert and collectively stand in prayer, imploring God to lift the plague. Even though such a practice had been recorded to have been undertaken periodically in the fourteenth century since the years of the Black Death, Ibn Ḥajar tells us it was controversial—so disputed, in fact, that the sultan invited the realm's preeminent scholars to rule on it, and a number issued competing opinions on its religious legitimacy and benefits.

For Ibn Ḥajar's part, he had found nothing in the Hadith, nor precedent from Islam's earliest generations, to support such a practice. He noted that while there was such a prayer for rain during times of drought, none existed for the plague. He added that not only did the practice lack religious grounding, it also seemed to lack efficacy. If anything, it appeared to have made the plague worse. He put into practice what he preached when he refused to appear by the Sultan al-Muʾayyad Shaykh's side during these processionals to the desert, despite the fact that he was politically very close to him and that they apparently viewed each other with mutual respect.

The need for the book became even more apparent in the wake of the 1430 outbreak, which was much more severe. By that point, Ibn Ḥajar had already made great headway on *The Divine Aid to Victory*, a work that addressed almost every aspect of the human experience and thus also included discussions of plague, medicine, martyrdom, contagion, death, prayer, patience and contemplation, the theological problem of evil and suffering, and many other issues that would have bearing on the themes he would treat in *Merits of the Plague*. In fact, Ibn Ḥajar himself tells us that he excerpted relevant passages from *The Divine Aid to Victory*, which may have given this book the gravitas, prestige, and distinction to attract a broader audience.

Whatever the motivations, the end result is a work whose central goal was the investigation and synthesis of the vast corpus of hadiths on the plague and the many dimensions of Muslim ethical, legal, theological, historical, and political discourses on disease, epidemics, and natural disasters more broadly. For the educated public, the book offered a practical guide to those responses to the plague that were securely rooted in the example of the Prophet and his Companions. At its core, it proposes a counterintuitive argument that is captured in rhyme by the book's full title, *Offering Aid on the Merits of the Plague* (*Badhl al-Māʿūn fī Faḍl al-Ṭaʿūn*): the plague presents an opportunity to practice patience and social care, allowing one to achieve merit or even martyrdom in the eyes of God.

Two features mark Ibn Ḥajar's scholarly method in *Merits of the Plague*: exhaustiveness and synthesis. As the consummate hadith scholar, Ibn Ḥajar was keen to locate all the hadiths and their variant forms that were potentially relevant to an issue at hand, such as the plague's etiology or whether one should flee a city afflicted by the plague. As a polymath, he referred to—and often quoted verbatim—the views of jurists, theologians, poets, scholars of medicine, and philosophers on the issue being addressed. Once having collected centuries of quotations on a given issue, he then identified and reconciled any differences between these sources. Sometimes contradictions presented themselves among different hadiths, with variant versions of the hadith creating a *Rashomon*-like effect, capturing the same event from multiple perspectives. At other times, differences emerged among scholars across various disciplines or between those scholars and the apparent meaning of a hadith. Ibn Ḥajar's primary goal was to sift through these contradictions and harmonize them. Rarely did he outright reject a hadith for source-critical reasons, or for a scholarly view, for that matter. Rather, he attempted to reconcile any differences between the sources—oftentimes to show that, in effect, the apparent contradiction was only an illusion.

Ibn Ḥajar was aware that his book would be read by specialists, too, and he was careful to make sure that it would not only pass muster with them, but would also elevate the quality of scholarship on the subject. Indeed, evidence from at least one manuscript, which is littered with corrections and additions in the margins, suggests that specialists in the hadith sciences made use of this book in their study circles in the decades after it began circulating.[26]

The book opens with a sequence of essential hadiths on the plague, each accompanied by a special kind of citation called an isnad: a series of names of the hadith's transmitters linking Ibn Ḥajar's source—typically an esteemed multivolume hadith collection—to one of Muhammad's Companions or wives who recalled hearing him utter a certain phrase or seeing him perform a certain act. Ibn Ḥajar did not take the veracity of these citations for granted, and he graded their reliability to be sound, weak, or fair by investigating the relative trustworthiness of the cited transmitters, and whether there are any corroborating reports or missing links in the isnad. Those hadiths whose authority were firmly established through this source-critical process became the foundation of Ibn Ḥajar's understanding of the plague; those that he considered weak or even erroneous could undermine his opponents if they had cited them in their arguments. Whatever role these narrative accounts played in Ibn Ḥajar's larger argument, they are compelling and valuable on their own terms, since they offer readers a glimpse of how early Muslims may have responded to epidemics during and just after the rise of Islam.[27]

The opening chapter also greets readers familiar with the Hebrew Bible with an account of Moses, Pharaoh, and the story of plagues that took place during Passover, as well as another involving the story of Moses, Balaam, and Zimri that tracks a similar version in the book of Numbers. Alongside the prophetic hadiths, these accounts are cited as historical evidence of the early origins of the plague and the way the plague was seen as a manifestation of God's wrath prior to the coming of Islam. Other figures from the Hebrew Bible and the New Testament—such as Adam and Eve, Noah, Ezekiel, and Jesus—appear later in the book to make a similar point. While it may strike some readers as odd to see a Muslim scholar citing such accounts reverently, given the fraught history among Muslims,

Christians, and Jews, readers new to this material should bear in mind that Adam, Moses, Noah, Jesus, and many other biblical characters appear in the Qur'an as prophets and are as integral to the Islamic tradition as they are to Judaism or Christianity.

In the next chapter, *Merits of the Plague* grapples with the various theories of the disease. Ibn Ḥajar weaves together medical sources, theological sources, and hadith literature in an attempt to define the plague, its causes, and its relation to other kinds of epidemics. The chapter begins by describing how the plague manifests itself on the surface of the body as well as in the internal organs. It describes and contests the concept of miasma—the notion that the plague contaminates the air as it rises from rotting corpses wounded on the battlefield—as one potential explanation of the plague. Ultimately, though, it establishes the authenticity of the hadiths that assert that the jinn—unseen spirits mentioned in the Qur'an—"pierce" the human body with unseen "pricks," which cause the buboes, sores, and pustules to form. The chapter concludes that recitation of Qur'anic chapters and supplicatory prayers can be legitimately invoked to repel jinn and thus the plague.

In establishing the idea that the plague is not contagious, and instead that it is caused by the "pricks of the jinn," Ibn Ḥajar does not see himself as being at odds with his time's medical account of the plague's etiology, which held "that the plague results from poisonous matter or a stirring up of blood or the flowing of it to a body part."[28] He argues, after all, that such an understanding does not exclude the jinn's pricks from leading to this chain of events in the blood and the body. He also takes pains to supplement his belief that the plague was caused by the "pricks of the jinn" with an empirical observation: The theories of contagion and miasma of his day—which did not understand the role of fleas in the transmission of the bubonic form of the plague—could not explain why we observe a man to be afflicted by buboes, while other members of his household appeared to be untouched by the disease. In the face of this apparent contradiction of the medical theory, the explanation that jinn were responsible for spreading the disease to select individuals appeared to line up better with the empirical observations.[29]

At the end of this chapter, Ibn Ḥajar offers a firsthand account of a chief adviser to the sultan who, after having been doubtful of the jinn's connection to the disease, claimed he heard the voices of invisible spirits plotting to strike plague upon an unsuspecting horse. This again suggests that his position, which was established in theory by the hadiths, was corroborated by observable practice.

Having established that the jinn are the proximate terrestrial cause of the plague—rather than person-to-person contagion—Ibn Ḥajar was prepared, in his third chapter, to answer the fundamental question raised by the pandemic: Why are both those who are innocent and those who are deserving of punishment killed by the plague? Part of his answer requires reframing the plague as an invisible spiritual battle between good and evil, in which jinn who believe in God pierce those deserving of punishment, and jinn who disobey God pierce the righteous of humankind. Like heroes of war, the righteous who die fighting bravely in God's path on the battlefield are rewarded with martyrdom. Even believing sinners who die of the plague are guaranteed martyrdom, though they may not attain the same level in paradise as the righteous martyrs.

A key piece of evidence for this third chapter, and indeed for the argument of the book, rests on a hadith that asserts that anyone "who stays in his home in patience and hopeful of heavenly reward, knowing that he shall not be struck with plague unless God has already inscribed such a fate for him" will be rewarded as a martyr. One indication of this hadith's importance is the amount of space Ibn Ḥajar devotes to exhaustively examining its variant versions in order to establish its credibility, something he does not do for all hadiths. Ibn Ḥajar's aim in this section is to establish just how attainable the heavenly rewards of martyrdom are for an ordinary person during times of plague. No extraordinary acts of bravery on the battlefield are required; rather, all that the Prophet asks of a believer is to remain in place and practice patience, remain hopeful of God's mercy, and cultivate acceptance of His decree.

Ibn Ḥajar also uses the third chapter to address other curiosities, contradictions, and interpretive problems that arise from certain hadiths, such as a famous one claiming that the plague "would never enter Medina's gates." If the plague truly represented a mercy for believers, why would God have prevented it from entering there? It is in reckoning with all of these questions, great and small, that Ibn Ḥajar comes closest to grappling with the meaning of suffering and mass death, and to treating the plague as a case study to gain new insight into the problem of evil.

The book's fourth chapter builds on this argument by enjoining believers not to flee from the plague, even though they may have a strong desire to do so. Once again, the strength of Ibn Ḥajar's case rests on a hadith that he believes reliably establishes that the Prophet called upon people to neither flee nor enter a place beset by plague. Ibn Ḥajar recognizes that many people, seized by fear of contagion, would be tempted to flee such a place, but he explains why such behavior is misguided: There is no contagion; rather, it is God who chooses who lives or dies. Not only will the plague follow those fleeing wherever they go, but also those who flee will leave behind their responsibility to tend to the sick and the weak, and to prepare burials for the dead. Meanwhile, those who cultivate patience, assist others, and remain in the afflicted city will be rewarded by God. It is in these moments that Ibn Ḥajar broadens his case beyond the fate of an individual and his relationship with God to encompass the well-being of society and the individual's responsibility toward maintaining communal welfare.

In the fifth chapter, the book enters the realm of what today we might call applied ethics, by addressing the moral and legal quandaries that arise as a consequence of the plague. If your town is struck by the plague, and death seems imminent, does that legally affect your ability to dispose of your wealth? What are the best practices for those who are afflicted and those treating them? The issue of contagion is again of great import here, and Ibn Ḥajar addresses the efficacy of social distancing, and whether congregational prayers in the desert specifically intended to repel the plague do more harm than good. At times, he shows he is aware that some of his most devoted readers may be in danger of taking his conclusions too far. For instance, if one can achieve the status of a martyr by dying of the plague, why not deliberately expose oneself to the disease? This chapter also offers readers a window into the world of medieval medical treatments, including rose oil, apple oil, bloodletting, cautery, and other surgical procedures.

The final chapter—technically an epilogue—is a vibrant and rich anthology of various literary and historical depictions of the plague. It offers a chronology of the plague from the time of the Prophet to Ibn Ḥajar's era and documents official registers of death counts that track the spread of the plague in various years and decades across history. Other sections within this chapter reproduce letters and relay firsthand accounts from witnesses in Damascus and Cairo, and characterize the political and religious attempts to manage the outbreak, as well as the struggles of ordinary people who bore the brunt of the burden and of death. In one revealing passage, Ibn Ḥajar describes how older men seemed to avoid death almost entirely, while countless women and younger people were casualties. These firsthand accounts offer a sober reminder that the burden of epidemics is not shared equally—not in the past, and certainly not now.

Ibn Ḥajar was recognized as a poet of some ability, and he collects here several prose poems on the plague, in order of what he judges to be their literary merit. He reproduces "Tidings of the Plague," the famous poem of Ibn al-Wardī, who witnessed the Black Death of 1347. The poem personifies the plague as an abuser, an incarnation of lust and unbridled male desire, and tracks "his" trail of devastation and harassment across various parts of the known world, from western China to Crimea to Egypt, as well as the local spread of the disease among smaller villages in Syria, locations that are gendered in Arabic with the feminine she/her/hers. Ibn al-Wardī's use of he/him/his pronouns to personify the plague thus not only amplifies the violence by imbuing it with a disturbing sexual dimension but also creates some productive ambiguity, since

God is also referred to with male pronouns. At the heart of the poem, this provocative tension rises to the fore: Is the plague a villainous serpent, or a meritorious manifestation of God's will and mercy? "Tidings of the Plague" explores this blurry boundary between a seemingly all-powerful plague and an all-powerful God.

Not only a striking and powerful response to the Black Death, "Tidings" is also didactic, unsparing in its social criticism, sums up many of the legal and theological points Ibn Ḥajar argues for in *Merits of the Plague*, and does so with gusto and great wit. It lampoons both the pious villagers spared by the plague—believing themselves to be more righteous than their neighbors—as well as the wayward urban elite who ate a comical diet of onions, vinegar, and sardines, hoping that it would somehow rid them of the disease. One could imagine that, when *Merits of the Plague* was read aloud among study circles and larger audiences, this epilogue would have functioned to recapitulate the main points of the book in an accessible and memorable way.

The book concludes with a particularly fitting final hadith. It describes the scene of a great hadith scholar stricken with the disease, with students surrounding him on his deathbed. One student asks another to recite the hadith in which the Prophet instructs that the dying should be prompted to utter the phrase "There is no god but God," since "He whose last words are 'There is no god but God' enters paradise." The student is unable to bring himself to complete the recollection of the hadith, but then the master, in the agonizing throes of death, lifts his head to recite the hadith before expiring. The story is a perfect example of how one, in Ibn Ḥajar's mind, could die of plague while fighting in God's path. It also demonstrates how the isnad was not simply a citation history that established the soundness of a hadith but also a rope with which one could tie oneself ever closer to the Prophet and thus closer to God. And it is a perfect reversal of the hadith itself, which enjoins the living to remind the dying—not the dying to remind the living—that "There is no god but God."

Merits of the Plague was read and reread by learned Muslim audiences throughout the Mamluk and Ottoman periods, by both hadith specialists and broader audiences seeking a guide for the perplexed. Ibn Ḥajar's students—among them al-Suyūṭī (d. 1505) and Zakariyyā al-Anṣārī (d. 1520)—abridged and adapted it for different audiences, simplifying some aspects of Ibn Ḥajar's form, choosing different emphases, and adding new material as well.[30]

The book made its way to Europe perhaps as early as the late sixteenth century; for instance, the Royal Library at the Escorial, in Spain, likely acquired an early copy of the work at this time, or perhaps in the early seventeenth century. In 1760, Miguel Casiri, a librarian at the Escorial, gave the author and his volume a Latin name: the *Obedientia et Utilitas* of "Ahmad Ascalonensis," commonly known as "Ebn Hagiar."[31] Casiri's eighteenth-century bibliographical notes suggest that he saw the work—which he classified as a "tractatus dogmatico-historico de peste"—as having two key points: one should not flee from the plague, and those who died of plague were considered martyrs.

While never translated into a European language, *Merits of the Plague* was republished in the 1990s in two separate editions in Arabic. In the era of the coronavirus, it reappeared in public discourse among Muslims, as major news and media outlets, such as IslamOnline and Hawiya Press, published features on it, and video commentaries on it by Muslim scholars and students cropped up on YouTube.

Western scholars of infectious diseases in Islamic contexts have found interest in this work as well, and their assessments of it have changed over time. In the 1970s, Manfred Ullmann said that it represented the writings of an unenlightened religious scholar in which "bigotry and magic dissolve rational reflection with amulets and prayers."[32] Since then, recent scholars, influenced by Michael Dols's *The Black Death in the Middle East*, have been more deferential to Ibn Ḥajar's achievement, viewing it as a crystallization of the orthodox Islamic position on the plague.[33] Jaqueline Sublet, who summarized the work in

French, similarly saw its value as a reflection of mainstream Islamic jurisprudence of the time.[34]

More recently, Justin Stearns has pushed back against this notion, arguing that Ibn Ḥajar was just one voice—albeit an influential one—among many diverse and competing Muslim voices within the dynamic intellectual discourse on disease in the Islamic world. For instance, several prominent medieval and early modern Muslim scholars, contra Ibn Ḥajar, defended the idea that diseases like the plague were contagious and instructed audiences to flee the plague accordingly. Among them were Ibn al-Khaṭīb (d. 1374) and Ibn Khātima (d. 1369), whose writings on the plague circulated in North Africa and the Islamic West, as well as al-Bidlīsī (d. 1520), a respected scholar who found alternating employment in the Ottoman, Safavid, and Mamluk courts, and whose work was later cited by modern Muslim scholars in favor of quarantines, a separate issue but one related to the matter of contagion.[35] No classic emerges in a vacuum, then, and while *Merits of the Plague* represents an influential Muslim response to the plague, it had meaningful competition and vocal interlocutors.

Acknowledging the richness and diversity of plague treatises in Islamic thought brings us to a related point best articulated by Nükhet Varlik, who, echoing the work of Lawrence Conrad, argued that Ibn Ḥajar's work is best understood as part of a long tradition of plague treatises with its own genre conventions and literary expectations. While *Merits of the Plague* may stand out in terms of its stature and influence, Varlik sees it as an invitation to study the evolution of this broader and collective practice of writing and transmitting plague treatises.[36]

In his biography of Ibn Ḥajar, Kevin Jaques argued that "Ibn Hajar could not accept the idea, prevalent in his day, that God punished sin through the plague," a position that would help him reckon with the death of three of his own daughters, two of whom were young children.[37] While Ibn Ḥajar saw the plague as a mercy for most Muslims, the story, as we have seen, was more complicated. He did think the plague could be thought of as a punishment for those who disbelieved, or for those Muslims who were gravely disobedient. Indeed, it is this tension—that the plague can offer the opportunity for both recompense *and* retribution—that animates the book.

The genius of Ibn Ḥajar's work, then, lies in its ability to grapple with this apparent contradiction, positing, through the compilation of hadiths, history, literature, and scholarly opinions from centuries past, a novel argument: it is precisely at one of history's darkest moments, when God appears most punishing and capricious, and death invades every home, that God's mercy is most expansive.

JOEL BLECHER *and* MAIRAJ SYED

NOTES

1. Lester K. Little, "Plague Historians in Lab Coats," *Past & Present*, 213/1 (2011): 267–90; Nahyan Fancy and Monica Green, "Plague and the Fall of Baghdad (1258)," *Medical History*, 65/2 (2021): 157–77.
2. Ebrahim Moosa, "Saudi Arabia Must Suspend the Hajj," *New York Times*, April 27, 2020.
3. Michael Dols, "Plague in Early Islamic History," *Journal of the American Oriental Society*, 94/3 (1974): 371–83.
4. Monica Green, "The Four Black Deaths," *American Historical Review*, 125/5 (2020): 1600–631.
5. Michael Dols, *The Black Death in the Middle East* (Princeton: Princeton University Press, 1977), 66.
6. Dols, *The Black Death*, 143–92, 255–80; Stuart Borsch, "Plague Depopulation and Irrigation Decay in Medieval Egypt," *The Medieval Globe*, 1/1 (2014): 125–56.
7. The complete anecdote describing this affair, preserved by Ibn Ḥajar, has been translated in the appendix of this volume. See Ibn Ḥajar al-ʿAsqalānī, *Inbāʾ al-ghumr bi-anbāʾ al-ʿumr*, ed. Ḥasan Ḥabashī (Cairo: Majlis al-Aʿla lʾil-Shuʿun al-Islāmiyya, 1969–1998): 3:438.
8. See the appendix to this volume, "From Ibn Ḥajar's 'Journal of the Plague Years.'"
9. Ibn Ḥajar al-ʿAsqalānī, *Inbāʾ al-ghumr bi-anbāʾ al-ʿumr*, 4:71;

Aḥmad ibn ʿAlī al-Maqrīzī, *Kitāb al-Sulūk li-Maʿrifat Duwal al-Mulūk*, ed. Muhammad ʿAbd al-Qadir ʿAṭā (Beirut: Dār al-Kutub al-ʿIlmiyya, 1997): 7:354.

10. For an account of one such multifaith processional, see the appendix to this volume, "From Ibn Ḥajar's 'Journal of the Plague Years.'" In European countries bordering the Mediterranean, attacks on religious minorities were rarer, and practices of blame casting and supplication to God parallel those we find in Mamluk Cairo. See Abigail Agresta, "From Purification to Protection: Plague Response in Late Medieval Valencia," *Speculum*, 95/2 (2020): 371–95. On the scapegoating of the Jews in Germany during the Black Death, see Samuel Cohn, "The Black Death and the Burning of Jews," *Past and Present*, 196 (2007): 3–36.
11. Dols, *The Black Death*, 121–42.
12. Justin K. Stearns, *Infectious Ideas: Contagion in Premodern Islamic and Christian Thought in the Western Mediterranean* (Baltimore: Johns Hopkins University Press, 2011).
13. Michael Christopher Low, "Empire and the Hajj: Pilgrims, Plagues, and Pan-Islam under British Surveillance, 1865–1908," *International Journal of Middle East Studies*, 40/2 (2008), 269–90; idem, *Imperial Mecca: Ottoman Arabia and the Indian Ocean Ḥajj* (New York: Columbia University Press, 2020), 117–66.
14. Nükhet Varlik, "'Oriental Plague' or Epidemiological Orientalism? Revisiting the Plague Episteme of the Early Modern Mediterranean," *Plague and Contagion in the Islamic Mediterranean* (Amsterdam: ARC, Amsterdam University Press, 2017): 57–88.
15. These opinions are documented in Harvard's Shariasource collection of Muslim legal responsa (*fatwā*s) to COVID-19; see "Mapping COVID-19 Fatwas," *Islamic Law Blog*, https://islamiclaw.blog/2020/05/04/mapping-covid-19-fatwas/, accessed February 16, 2022.
16. Biographical material is culled from Shams al-Dīn al-Sakhāwī's *al-Jawāhir wa'l-durar* (Beirut: Dār Ibn Ḥazm, 1999), a work on the life of Ibn Ḥajar written by his closest student, and Ibn Ḥajar's own autobiography, which is now available in English: Kristen Brustad et al., *Interpreting the Self: Autobiography in the Arabic Literary Tradition,* ed. Dwight Reynolds (Berkeley: University of California Press, 2001), 81–84. See also Sabri Kawash, "Ibn Ḥajar al-[ʿ]Asqalānī (1372–1449 A.D.): A Study of

the Background, Education, and Career of a[n] ʿĀlim in Egypt," PhD diss., Princeton University, 1970; and Kevin Jaques, *Ibn Hajar* (New Delhi: Oxford University Press, 2009).

17. Brustad et al., *Interpreting the Self: Autobiography in the Arabic Literary Tradition,* 81–84.
18. Brustad et al., *Interpreting the Self*, 81–84.
19. Yossef Rapoport, "Ibn Ḥağar al-ʿAsqalānī, His Wife, Her Slave-Girl: Romantic Triangles and Polygamy in 15th Century Cairo," *Annales Islamologiques* 47 (2013): 332–33.
20. See *Merits of the Plague (this volume)*, 222.
21. See *Merits of the Plague (this volume)*, 224.
22. Rapoport, "Ibn Ḥağar al-ʿAsqalānī, His Wife, Her Slave-Girl," 346.
23. Joel Blecher, *Said the Prophet of God: Hadith Commentary across a Millennium* (Oakland: University of California Press, 2018), 53–54.
24. Ibn Ḥajar, *Inbāʾ al-ghumr bi-anbāʾ al-ʿumr*, 4:224.
25. See *Merits of the Plague (this volume)*, 1.
26. See Gowaart Van Den Bossche's description of *Badhl al-Māʿūn fī Fawāʾid al-Ṭāʿūn*, Egyptian National Library and Archives, MS Ḥadīth Taymūr, 198, https://ihodp.ugent.be/bah/mml01%3A000000386#collapse-rdfextrashowrdf, accessed February 10, 2021.
27. For more on this, see Stearns, *Infectious Ideas*, 163–64; Josef van Ess, *Der Fehltritt des Gelehrten* (Heidelberg: C. Winter, 2001), 125–26.
28. See *Merits of the Plague (this volume)*, 22–23.
29. In spite of this important disagreement, readers should keep in mind that the Galenic medical tradition was not necessarily in conflict with religious works like Ibn Ḥajar's *Merits of the Plague*; on the contrary, generations of hadith scholars during this period had attempted to harmonize the Greek tradition with the hadiths, synthesizing the two in a new genre they called "prophetic medicine." Indeed, in chapter five of this book, Ibn Ḥajar even takes some physicians to task for failing to take up Galenic practices like bloodletting to treat the plague. For more on this subject, see the translator's introduction to Ibn al-Qayyim al-Jawziyya, *Medicine of the Prophet*, trans. Penelope Johnstone (Islamic Texts Society, 1998), xxiii–xxxii; Irmeli Perho, *The Prophet's Medicine: A Creation of the Muslim Traditionalist Scholars* (Helsinki: Kokemäki, 1995).

30. Jalāl al-Dīn al-Suyūṭī, *Mā rawāhu al-wāʿūn fī akhbār al-ṭāʿūn* (Damascus: Dār al-Qalam, 1997); for Zakariyyā al-Anṣārī's *Tuḥfat al-rāghibīn fī bayān amr al-ṭawāʿīn*, see Hans Daiber, "Plague and Consolation in a Newly Discovered Text by Zakariyāʾ al-Anṣārī (d. 926/1520)," in *From the Greeks to the Arabs and Beyond*, 3 vols. (Leiden: Brill, 2021), 3:289–390.
31. Casiri's Latin name for *Merits* might translate to "Obedience and Benefit," and his classification would be "a religio-historical tract on the plague." See Miguel Casiri, *Bibliotheca Arabico-Hispana Escurialensis*, 2 vols. (Madrid: de Soto, 1760), I:522; s.v. "Ahmad Ascalonensis" in the index of volume II.
32. Manfred Ullmann, *Islamic Medicine* (Edinburgh: Edinburgh University Press, 1978), 96.
33. Dols, *The Black Death*, 8 and passim.
34. Jacqueline Sublet, "La peste prise aux rêts de la jurisprudence: Le traité d'Ibn Ḥağar al-'Asqalānī sur la peste," *Studia Islamica,* 33 (1971): 141–49.
35. Justin Stearns, "Public Health, the State, and Religious Scholarship Sovereignty in Idrīs al-Bidlīsī's Arguments for Fleeing the Plague," in *The Scaffolding of Sovereignty: Global and Aesthetic Perspectives on the History of a Concept*, ed. Zvi Benite, Stefanos Geroulanos, and Nicole Jerr (New York: Columbia University Press, 2017): 163–85.
36. Nükhet Varlik, "Between Local and Universal: Translating Knowledge in Early Modern Ottoman Plague Treati[s]es," in *Knowledge in Translation: Global Patterns of Scientific Exchange, 1000–1800 CE*, ed. Patrick Manning and Abigail Owen (Pittsburgh: University of Pittsburgh Press): 170–90.
37. Kevin Jaques, *Ibn Hajar* (New Delhi: Oxford University Press, 2009), 6.

Suggestions for Further Reading

EDITIONS

ʿAsqalānī, Ibn Ḥajar al-. *Badhl al-māʿūn fī faḍl al-ṭāʿūn*. Edited by Aḥmad ʿIṣām ʿAbd al-Qādir al-Kātib. Riyadh: Dār al-ʿĀṣima, 1991.

———. *Badhl al-māʿūn fī faḍl al-ṭāʿūn*. Edited by Abū Ibrahīm Kaylānī Muḥammad Khalīfa. Cairo: Dār al-Kutub al-Athariyya, 1993.

———. *Inbāʾ al-ghumr bi-anbāʾ al-ʿumr*. Edited by Ḥasan Ḥabashī. 4 vols. Cairo: Majlis al-Aʿlā li al-Shuʾūn al-Islāmiyya, 1969–1998.

———. *Inbāʾ al-ghumr bi-anbāʾ al-ʿumr*. Edited by Muḥammad Khān. Beirut: Dār al-Kutub al-ʿIlmiyya. Hyderabad: Maṭbaʿa Majlis Dāʾira al-Maʿārif al-ʿUthmāniyya, 1986.

PLAGUE, PANDEMICS, AND ISLAMIC HISTORY

Barker, Hannah. "Laying the Corpses to Rest: Grain, Embargoes, and *Yersinia pestis* in the Black Sea, 1346–1348." *Speculum*, 96/1 (2021): 97–126.

Borsch, Stuart J. *The Black Death in Egypt and England: A Comparative Study*. Austin: University of Texas Press, 2005.

Borsch, Stuart J., and Tarek Sabraa. "Plague Mortality in Late Medieval Cairo: Quantifying the Plague Outbreaks of 833/1430 and 864/1460." *Mamluk Studies Review*, 19 (2016): 57–90.

Conrad, Lawrence I. "Arabic Plague Chronologies and Treatises: Social and Historical Factors in the Formation of a Literary Genre." *Studia Islamica*, 54 (1981): 51–93.

———. "*Ṭāʿūn* and *Wabāʾ*: Conceptions of Plague and Pestilence in Early Islam." *Journal of the Economic and Social History of the Orient*, 25 (1982): 268–307.

Dols, Michael W. *The Black Death in the Middle East.* Princeton: Princeton University Press, 1977.

———. "Plague in Early Islamic History." *Journal of the American Oriental Society*, 94/3 (1974): 371–83.

———. "Ibn al-Wardī's *Risālah al-Nabā' 'an al-Wabā'*: A Translation of a Major Source for the History of the Black Death in the Middle East." In *Near Eastern Numismatics, Iconography, Epigraphy and History: Studies in Honor of George C. Miles*, edited by Dickran K. Kouymjian. Beirut: American University of Beirut, 1974: 443–55.

Fancy, Nahyan, and Monica Green. "Plague and the Fall of Baghdad (1258)." *Medical History*, 65/2 (2021): 157–77.

Green, Monica H. "Taking 'Pandemic' Seriously: Making the Black Death Global." In *Pandemic Disease in the Medieval World: Rethinking the Black Death*, edited by Monica Green. Kalamazoo, Mich.: Arc Humanities Press, 2015, 27–62.

Low, Michael C. "Empire and the Hajj: Pilgrims, Plagues, and Pan-Islam under British Surveillance, 1865–1908." *International Journal of Middle East Studies*, 40/2 (2008), 269–90.

Portmann, Peter E., and Emilie Savage-Smith. *Medieval Islamic Medicine.* Edinburgh: Edinburgh University Press, 2010.

Stearns, Justin K. *Infectious Ideas: Contagion in Premodern Islamic and Christian Thought in the Western Mediterranean.* Baltimore: Johns Hopkins University Press, 2011.

Tagliacozzo, Eric. "Hajj in the Time of Cholera: Pilgrim Ships and Contagion from Southeast Asia to the Red Sea." In *Global Muslims in the Age of Steam and Print Book*, edited by James L. Gelvin and Nile Green. Berkeley: University of California Press, 2013, 103–20.

Ullmann, Manfred. *Islamic Medicine.* Edinburgh: Edinburgh University Press, 1978.

Varlik, Nükhet. "Between Local and Universal: Translating Knowledge in Early Modern Ottoman Plague Treati[s]es." In *Knowledge in Translation: Global Patterns of Scientific Exchange, 1000–1800 CE*, edited by Patrick Manning and Abigail Owen. Pittsburgh: University of Pittsburgh Press, 2018.

———, ed. *Plague and Contagion in the Islamic Mediterranean.* Kalamazoo, Mich.: Arc Humanities Press, 2017.

———. *Plague and Empire in the Early Modern World: The Ottoman Experience, 1347–1600.* Cambridge: Cambridge University Press, 2015.

IBN ḤAJAR AL-ʿASQALĀNĪ

Bauer, Thomas. "Ibn Ḥajar al-ʿAsqalānī, *Diwān*. Edited by Firdaws Nūr ʿAlī Ḥusayn (Madinat Naṣr: Dār al-Fikr al-ʿArabī, 1416/1996). pp. 358." *Mamluk Studies Review*, 4 (2000): 267–68.

———. "Ibn Ḥajar and the Arabic Ghazal of the Mamluk Age." In *Ghazal as World Literature I: Transformations of a Literary Genre*, edited by T. Bauer and A. Neuwirth. Beirut: Ergon Verlag Wu'rzburg in Kommission, 2005, 35–55.

Blecher, Joel. "Ḥadīth Commentary in the Presence of Students, Patrons, and Rivals: Ibn Ḥajar and *Ṣaḥīḥ Al-Bukhārī* in Mamluk Cairo." *Oriens*, 41, nos. 3/4 (2013): 261–87.

———. "Revision in the Manuscript Age: New Evidence of Early Versions of Ibn Ḥajar's *Fatḥ al-Bārī*." *Journal of Near Eastern Studies*, 76/1 (2017): 39–51.

Brustad, Kristen, Michael Cooperson, Jamal Elias, Nuha Khoury, Joseph Lowry, Nasser Rabbat, Dwight Reynolds, Devin Stewart, and Shawkat Toowara. *Interpreting the Self: Autobiography in the Arabic Literary Tradition*, ed. Dwight Reynolds. Berkeley: University of California Press, 2001.

Conrad, Lawrence I. "Ibn Ḥajar-ʿAsqalānī, Abū l-Faḍl Aḥmad Ibn ʿAlī, *Badhl al-ma'ūn fī faḍl al-ṭā'ūn*. Edited by Abū Ibrāhim Kaylānī Muhammad Khalīfa. Cairo, Dār al-kutub al-athariya, 1413/1993, pp. 246, no price given." *Medical History*, 39/3 (1995): 391–93.

Fadel, Mohammad. "Ibn Ḥajar's Hady al-Sārī: A Medieval Interpretation of the Structure of al-Bukhārī's *al-Jāmiʿ al-Ṣaḥīḥ*: Introduction and Translation." *Journal of Near Eastern Studies*, 54/3 (1995): 161–97.

Hassan, Mona. "Poetic Memories of the Prophet's Family: Ibn Ḥajar al-ʿAsqalānī's Panegyrics for the ʿAbbasid Sultan-Caliph of Cairo al-Mustaʿīn." *Journal of Islamic Studies*, 29/1 (2018): 1–24.

Jaques, Kevin. *Ibn Hajar*. New Delhi: Oxford University Press, 2009.

Kawash, Sabri. "Ibn Ḥajar al-[ʿ]Asqalānī (1372–1449 A.D.): A Study of the Background, Education, and Career of a[n] ʿĀlim in Egypt." PhD diss. Princeton: Princeton University, 1970.

Murad, Abdal Hakim. *Selections from the* Fatḥ al-Bārī *by Ibn Ḥajar al-ʿAsqalānī* (Cambridge: Muslim Academic Trust, 2000).

Rapoport, Yossef. "Ibn Ḥağar al-ʿAsqalānī, His Wife, Her Slave-Girl: Romantic Triangles and Polygamy in 15th-Century Cairo." *Annales Islamologiques*, 47 (2013): 327–52.

Rosenthal, Franz. "Ibn Ḥadjar al-ʿAsḳalānī." In *Encyclopaedia of Islam*, 2nd ed., edited by P. Bearman, Th. Bianquis, C. E. Bosworth, E. van Donzel, W. P. Heinrichs. Leiden: Brill, 1960–2007; online ed., 2012, http://dx.doi.org/10.1163/1573-3912_islam_SIM_3178.

Sublet, Jacqueline. "La peste prise aux rêts de la jurisprudence: Le traité d'Ibn Ḥağar al-ʿAsqalānī sur la peste." *Studia Islamica*, 33 (1971): 141–49.

A Note on the Translation

When it was first written, *Merits of the Plague* was intended to address a general audience of educated readers of its time. It includes a range of material to establish the credibility of its argument in the eyes of specialists in the hadith sciences. Our goal in translating it was to create an accessible reading experience that could reach as broad an audience as possible, while at the same time preserving some of the more technical information for those who are interested. Given that scholars will want to consult the source text in Arabic for themselves, we opted against a line-by-line simulation of an Arabic critical edition or a facsimile that aims to preserve every stray mark in the margins. In our view, such an effort would be doomed to come up short in preserving the spirit of the original.

To this end, we have made a number of editorial choices. First, we placed much of the citational and scholarly material that discusses the isnads in the endnotes, where specialists and those familiar with or interested in them can consult them. Had endnotes or footnotes been scholarly conventions in Ibn Ḥajar's day, we believe he would have made use of them in the way we have here. We further condensed, paraphrased, and often omitted material of this kind, notifying the reader in our endnotes when we have done so, and indicating to specialists where they can find a more detailed discussion or full isnads in the Arabic edition. Since his analysis of hadiths is a key a part of what distinguishes his work, we have preserved a handful of illustrative examples of Ibn Ḥajar's method of preserving, transmitting, and verifying isnads—and have often quoted Ibn Ḥajar's assessment of an isnad's authenticity so readers can get a taste of it. However, we have, by and large, spared the general-interest reader and students the task of wading through this highly technical material, which specialists will, in any event, prefer to consult in the original Arabic.

Second, we have omitted—typically without indicating that we have done so—any material where Ibn Ḥajar discusses the proper Arabic pronunciation of certain obscure words or proper names, or any grammatical or lexical points that were not pertinent to the argument. We have also omitted all of Ibn Ḥajar's end-of-chapter glossaries, which would serve little use to modern readers (although we have included a glossary and chronology of our own).

Third, we have clarified phrases or pronouns by making explicit a word or phrase that was clearly implied by the context. Typically, scholars will include these kinds of explanatory phrases in brackets or parentheses to indicate that they are not technically found in the source text. However, in order to facilitate the reading experience, we have discarded such conventions. Likewise, certain conventions that come across idiomatically in Arabic—such as the use of a double negative to indicate specification or exclusion—have been rephrased to sound more natural in English.

Fourth, while we left many of the original headings and subheadings intact, we adapted others to better capture the point under discussion or to more clearly introduce the subject of the section at hand. Ibn Ḥajar often paraphrased or previewed his argument in his headings, making some headings the length of one or two sentences. Since such subheadings would appear highly unusual for readers accustomed to modern English literary conventions, we have moved them from the headings into the opening sentence of the chapter. In rare cases, we even added a simple explanatory title where Ibn Ḥajar had only "Section."

We have also created a separate section for the epilogue—technically the *khatm* or closing section of the book—which printed editions have typically included as part of the fifth chapter. This is a more accurate representation of the original manuscript form.

Fifth, while we have left a handful of pious formulae such as "God, the Exalted," "May God be pleased with them," and "peace and blessings upon him" in certain passages for emphasis, we have removed them in most cases to maintain a smoothness of flow in English that emulates the unhesitating feel of the original Arabic. Modern Arabic editions of this text have tried to increase their concision in this regard by deploying various symbols, such as ﷺ as a glyph form of "peace and blessings upon him" (the formula that was present in the early manuscripts of this text following mention of the Prophet Muhammad). Again, to facilitate clarity for the widest possible audience and to maintain a visual uniformity in English that emulates the visual uniformity of the original, we have chosen not to include this modern symbol. Nevertheless, readers should be aware that these pious formulae would have been fundamental to the religiosity of the author and his Muslim audiences generally. They were also a basic element of the aural rhythm of the original, and would not have been perceived to burden or interrupt the attention of readers in Arabic.

Sixth, when Ibn Ḥajar cites titles of books, we translated them. Place names are given in transliterated Arabic except for commonly known regions and locations (e.g., Mecca, Baghdad, Egypt, India). Similarly, historical figures known to Western readers—Jesus, Noah, Avicenna—appear in their Latinized form, while others (Ibn al-Qayyim, al-Subkī, al-Bukhārī) retain an Arabic form. Long names of authorities have been shortened and standardized, typically without honorifics. Now that the term "isnad" is listed in English dictionaries, including the popular *Merriam-Webster Unabridged* dictionary, we have dispensed with the diacritics and employ "isnad" rather than the transliterated "isnād." The words "ibn" and "bint," which appear in many Arabic names, mean "son of" and "daughter of," respectively. Likewise, "Abū" and "Umm" mean "father of" and "mother of." The early generation of Muslims who knew Muḥammad are referred to as "the Companions," capitalized, as are the following generation, "the Successors." Dates are given according to the Islamic Calendar, with the Gregorian equivalents in parentheses.

For quotations from the Qur'an, we have adapted several translations—in particular, Muhammad Asad's *The Message of the Qur'an* and Wahiduddin Khan's *The Qur'an*, edited by Farida Khanam. For transliteration, we have relied largely on the standard conventions of the *International Journal of Middle East Studies*. Abbreviations we use frequently: *EI1*, to indicate *The Encyclopedia of Islam*, 1st edition, edited by M. Th. Houtsma, T. W. Arnold, R. Basset, and R. Hartmann (Leiden: Brill, 1913–1936); *EI2*, to indicate *The Encyclopedia of Islam*, 2nd edition, edited by P. Bearman, Th. Bianquis, C. E. Bosworth, E. van Donzel, and W. P. Heinrichs (Leiden: Brill, 1960–2007); *AEL*, to indicate E. W. Lane's *Arabic-English Lexicon*, 2 vols. (London: Williams and Norgate, 1863); and *BM*, to indicate *Badhl al-māʿūn fī faḍl al-ṭāʿūn*, edited by Aḥmad ʿIṣām ʿAbd al-Qādir al-Kātib (Riyadh: al-Mamlaka al-ʿArabīyya al-Saʿūdīyya: Dār al-ʿĀṣima, 1991). In general, we relied on Aḥmad ʿIṣām ʿAbd al-Qādir al-Kātib's 1991 Arabic edition of this text. Al-Kātib consulted several early manuscript versions of the text at libraries in Aleppo, Damascus, and Istanbul—including one from the Sulaymaniyah library that was dated to the summer of 1448, just months before Ibn Ḥajar's death—and included a useful source-critical apparatus in the footnotes.[1] We strongly prefer al-Kātib's edition to Abū Ibrahīm Kaylānī Muḥammad Khalīfa's 1993 edition; the latter, as Lawrence Conrad pointed out, suffers from numerous problems and is not adequate as a critical edition (nor does it pretend to be).[2] While the pandemic prevented us from traveling into the archives throughout the bulk of our writing process, we did sometimes consult a digitized version of a manuscript copied in 1491, four decades after Ibn Ḥajar's death, held by the Royal Library at the Escorial (MS Madrid, El Escorial, Derenbourg no. 1510; Casiri no. MDV). This helped clarify any lingering textual issues, and the Escorial manuscript represents a version of the text that al-Kātib did not consult. If we came across any minor errors or disagreed with al-Kātib's interpretation, we made the appropriate changes in our translation.

We have also added an appendix of excerpts drawn from Ibn Ḥajar's chronicle accounts of the plague, which include descriptions of the death of his own children, and of his being struck by what he inferred was the plague near the end of his life; we have titled the appendix "Ibn Ḥajar's 'Journal of the Plague Years,'" after Daniel Defoe's famous (but fictional) account. The excerpts here have been drawn from Ibn Ḥajar's chronicle *Inbāʾ al-ghumr bi-anbāʾ al-ʿumr* (Tidings of the Abundance in the News of the Ages), and we relied primarily on the Arabic printed edition of this work, edited by Ḥasan Ḥabashī, 4 vols. (Cairo: Majlis al-Aʿlā li-ʾl-Shuʿūn al-Islāmiyya, 1969–1998), consulting Muḥammad Khān's 1986 edition as well.

A NOTE ON THE TRANSLATION OF IBN AL-WARDĪ'S "TIDINGS OF THE PLAGUE"

In the epilogue of *Merits of the Plague*, Ibn Ḥajar includes a famous poem by Ibn al-Wardī (d. 749/1349), "Risālat al-Nabāʾ ʿan al-Wabāʾ" ("Tidings of the Plague").[3] In 1974, Michael Dols offered a literal rendering of the poem in a well-hidden and heavily annotated academic article, treating it as a key historical source for the spread of the plague.[4] But since Ibn Ḥajar appreciated it more for its literary qualities, the translation offered here represents a first attempt at a literary translation of this work into modern English, with appropriate liberties taken in several passages to preserve the poetic spirit of the original.

The poem relies heavily on allusions to the Qur'an, clichés, and quotations from the pantheon of well-known Arabic poetry. The effect of these allusions is difficult to convey without "Englishing" the text, to borrow a term from Michael Cooperson's *Impostures*, by quoting, for example, the King James Bible or lines from the English literary canon.[5] Our translation of "Tidings" solves this problem by relying on literary devices and phrasings drawn from the canon of classical rhetoric that are well represented in English literature, as if to create the feeling of having made an allusion without actually having made one. Close readers may find some actual allusions hidden here as well, with certain lines and forms calling to mind the likes of Dylan Thomas, Thomas Moore, William Blake, and Gertrude Stein. In keeping with Ibn al-Wardī's clarity, this translation has tended to favor crisp, single-syllable Saxon words rather than Latinate ones. The favoring of Saxon diction and heavy caesuras also faintly echoes *Beowulf*, an apt allusion given that the plague terrorizes mankind as Grendel did, a monster "with God's wrath laden."

Our translation of "Tidings" also retains the original Arabic pronouns for the plague (he/him/his) and the cities (she/her/hers). While Dols's 1974 translation used gender-neutral pronouns to refer to both places and plague (it/its), the pronoun choices we made here are truer to Ibn al-Wardī's personification of the plague, creating a text that is both more accurate and livelier. As we discussed in the introduction, making the plague gender-neutral would also completely obscure some of the clear analogizing of the plague to unbridled male desire and conceal the provocative tension between an all-powerful God and a seemingly all-powerful disease.

The poem is essentially an epitome of Ibn al-Wardī's chronicle account of the plague expressed in a common form of rhyming prose-poetry, which in Arabic is called sajʿ. Ibn al-Wardī's style is also preoccupied with wordplay and heavy end rhyme—rhetorical flourishes that are natural in Arabic but not English; to capture the effect of this wordplay more naturally, we deployed other devices, like off-rhyme, alliteration, and assonance. The translation also discards the traditional forms of rhyme and meter or blank verse in favor of a syllabic form with a variable foot: lines are limited to three to eight syllables, and occasionally break that rule for effect. This works for sajʿ, since that form is also variable in terms of line length and has no regular meter.

Concerning the indentations and formatting, early drafts omitted indentations and justified each stanza to the left, but the text failed to capture the motion and agitation at the center of the narrative: the plague's devastation as it traveled across the known world. Our solution was to first indent the poem in triads, but then to center-justify the text, creating an off-kilter, asymmetrical, and almost slithering effect. This is fitting, as the serpent appears and reappears in the poem as a metaphor for the plague.* The visual likewise calls to mind a miasmic smog of corrupt air as it drifts through the countryside.

To counterbalance these off-kilter stanzas, when Ibn al-Wardī quotes from the Qur'an or from the literary canon, we have placed them in italics, and centered them without indenting them in triads. When he is in his didactic mode, we have centered the stanzas, but left them unitalicized. These stanzas' visual symmetry signal that they are quotations and teachings that can be relied upon, terra firma amid a turbulent sea.

It is a distinct pleasure to be able to thank the many colleagues, friends, and family who assisted us in the making of this book, through both their encouragement and help. We would like to thank, first, Elias Muhanna, whose edition of Nuwayri's *Ultimate Ambition in the Arts of Erudition* carved a path for our book and offered a perfect model as we made our way. We would also like to thank, in particular, the following colleagues who offered us advice and material suggestions as we stumbled over the obstacles we encountered along the way: Sibtain Abidi, Abigail Agresta, Michael Cooperson, Nathaniel Deutsch, Muhammad Fadel, Nahyan Fancy, Steven Hopkins, Paul Love, Justin Stearns, Nükhet Varlik, Lev Weitz, and the participants of the working group on History of Infectious Disease in the Islamicate World, co-organized by Monica Green. We also thank the Institute for Middle East Studies at The George Washington University and the University of California,

*Michael Dols remarks in his study of the poem that the serpent was symbolically associated with the plague at the time; "Ibn al-Wardī's Risāla," 452, n. 55.

Davis, for providing funding for our publication-related expenses. We would like to thank The George Washington University history majors who enrolled in "The Plague in Islamic History" seminar in the fall of 2020—in particular, Laruen Kiker, Yosua Siagian, and Mark Thomas-Patterson; their thoughtful engagement with the material helped improve this book's introduction. We tip our cap to Marcos Chin for his creativity and inspiration in capturing the spirit of *Merits* in his cover illustration. Our cartographer, Bill Nelson, provided our maps. At Penguin, our editor, John Siciliano, has been an exemplar of patience as we sent him news of delay upon delay—and we are grateful for his capacious imagination and willingness to help this volume become a Penguin Classic. We also thank Marissa Davis and our production editor, Jennifer Tait, who helped transform an unvarnished Word doc into a polished printed book made of paper, ink, and glue. We would also like to thank the engineers of the GIPHY app, who provided tremendous entertainment as we text-messaged one another about our progress. Lastly, we thank our families for allowing us to spend many weekends and weeknights glued to our computer screens, translating Arabic.

Mairaj would like to thank his parents for their lifelong support, encouragement, and enduring love. He dedicates this work to them. He would like to thank his children, Ibrahim and Mariam, for making life joyous and interesting. He would like to especially acknowledge his wife, Erum Abbasi, for the constancy of her assurance, humor, and love. Finally, he would like to express gratitude to God, the source of all being, and send salutations to the Prophet Muhammad, may peace and blessings be upon him.

Joel would like to thank the love and support of his parents, Marc and Sharon, who purchased him his first Penguin Classic—an edition of Beowulf in Old English, with a Blake print on the cover. He thanks his brothers, Jacob and Ian, for both their friendship and their cutting wits. He thanks his wife and partner, Summer, whose serenity and perspective grounded him during the darkest days of the pandemic. He dedicates this book to two little persons who helped in their own ways: his daughter, Aria, and her baby brother, Hawthorn, who was born in the middle of it all.

NOTES

1. See *BM*, 52.
2. Lawrence Conrad, "Ibn Ḥajar-'Asqalānī, Abū l-Faḍl Aḥmad Ibn 'Alī, *Badhl al-ma'ūn fī faḍl al-ṭā'ūn*," *Medical History*, 39/3 (1995): 391–93.
3. Ibn al-Wardī was, like many Muslim scholars of his age, including Ibn Ḥajar, a kind of polymath: a poet, litterateur, chronicler, grammarian, and legal scholar. He was born in Maʿarrat al-Nuʿmān, a village in northern Syria, the same birthplace as another celebrated figure of the Arabic literary canon, Abū al-ʿAlāʾ al-Maʿarrī (d. 449/1058). He studied in Ḥamā, Damascus, and Aleppo, where he died in 749/1349 of the same plague he depicts in "Tidings of the Plague" and his chronicle account. That small villages and urban centers in Syria and Egypt receive the lion's share of his attention tracks with his own biography and social horizon within the Mamluk Sultanate. S.v. "Ibn al-Wardī," *El* 1 (Ben Cheneb, M.).
4. Michael Dols, "Ibn al-Wardī's *Risālah al-Nābaʾ ʿan al-Wabāʾ*: A Translation of a Major Source for the History of the Black Death in the Middle East," in *Near Eastern Numismatics, Iconography, Epigraphy and History: Studies in Honor of George C. Miles*, ed. Dickran K. Kouymjian (Beirut: American University of Beirut, 1974), 443–55.
5. Al-Ḥarīrī, *Impostures: Fifty Rogue Tales Translated Fifty Ways*, trans. Michael Cooperson (New York: New York University Press, 2021), l–li.

Chronology

541–549	Plague of Justinian, beginning of the first plague pandemic.
632	Death of the Prophet Muhammad.
638	Plague of ʿAmwās in Syria, thought to be a recurrent wave of the Justinian Plague; the outbreak occurs during the reigns of the early caliphs.
1258	Mongols lay siege to Baghdad and other cities in the Middle East, seeding plague reservoirs that spark the second plague pandemic, commonly known as the Black Death.
1349	The Black Death, known to Ibn Ḥajar as the Great Plague, decimates populations across the Middle East, North Africa, Europe, and Asia.
February 28, 1372	Ibn Ḥajar al-ʿAsqalānī is born in Cairo. His mother, Tujjār al-Ziftāwī, dies soon after, likely within a year.
December 17, 1375	Ibn Ḥajar is fully orphaned after his father dies of an illness.
December 1376	A powerful and wealthy spice merchant, Zakī al-Dīn al-Kharrūbī, becomes Ibn Ḥajar's principal guardian.
1382–1412	Reigns of Sultan Barqūq and his son, Nāṣir Faraj.

1383	Ibn Ḥajar accompanies al-Kharrūbī to Mecca for business and pilgrimage, and studies hadith literature for the first time.
February 1385	Al-Kharrūbī dies, and Ibn Ḥajar enters the care, in Alexandria, of Ibn al-Qattān, a man of learning who introduces Ibn Ḥajar to historical literature as well as notable scholars of the time.
1393–1406	Ibn Ḥajar studies the hadith sciences intensively with scholarly luminaries in Egypt, Syria, Yemen, and the Ḥijaz.
May 1396	Ibn Ḥajar is married to Uns ʿAbd al-Karīm ibn Aḥmad, the daughter of the inspector of the army, a high office in the Mamluk Empire.
March 1400	Ibn Ḥajar's first child is a born—a daughter, Zayn Khāṭūn.
1400–1401	Tamerlane makes incursions into Syria, besieging Damascus and rattling the Mamluks.
1403–1404	Famine exacerbates an inflationary crisis in Egypt.
March 1406	Ibn Ḥajar begins lecturing on hadiths at the Shaykhūniyya and several other colleges in Cairo.
1408–1409	Ibn Ḥajar is appointed mufti at the Palace of Justice in Cairo.
July 1410	Ibn Ḥajar is installed as a dean of academic and administrative affairs of Baybarsiyya college in Cairo.
1410–1411	Ibn Ḥajar begins work on the introduction to his magnum opus, *Fatḥ al-Bārī* (The Divine Aid to Victory), a commentary on al-Bukhārī's collection of authenticated hadiths.

May 29, 1412	The birth of Ibn Ḥajar's only son, born by a concubine previously possessed by his wife, Uns.
1412–1421	Reign of Sultan al-Mu'ayyad Shaykh.
Spring 1416	A severe outbreak of the plague strikes Cairo, and two of Ibn Ḥajar's daughters die: Fāṭima (two years old) and Ghāliya (eleven years old). Ibn Ḥajar begins to compose a book on the plague, which he would later completely revise.
Spring 1419	Another outbreak of plague in Cairo, accompanied by a dramatic solar eclipse two weeks later.
1422–1438	Reign of Sultan Ashraf Barsbāy.
December 31, 1423	Ibn Ḥajar is appointed chief judge of Egypt and Syria, a position he holds intermittently for twenty-one years.
Winter 1430	Year of "The Great Extinction," the deadliest plague to strike Egypt since the Black Death. Ibn Ḥajar's eldest dies of the disease while pregnant, and he begins work on *Merits of the Plague*.
1433	Ibn Ḥajar marries Layla bint Maḥmūd ibn Tughān, later a subject of his love poetry.
Winter 1437	Plague strikes Egypt; Sultan Barsbāy bans most women from public spaces as a remedy.
1438–1453	Reign of Sultan Jaqmaq. The ban on women in public spaces comes to an end at the start of his reign.
January 24, 1439	Ibn Ḥajar celebrates the completion of his magnum opus, *Fatḥ al-Bārī* (The Divine Aid to Victory), excerpts of which were included in *Merits of the Plague*.

Spring 1444	Plague reoccurs in Egypt, and Ibn Ḥajar himself suffers from the bubonic form of the disease, but recovers.
August 26, 1448	Ibn Ḥajar is removed from the office of the chief judge of Egypt and Syria for the last time.
February 22, 1449	Amid the reoccurrence of plague, Ibn Ḥajar dies after battling an unknown illness for several months.

The World of *Merits of the Plague*

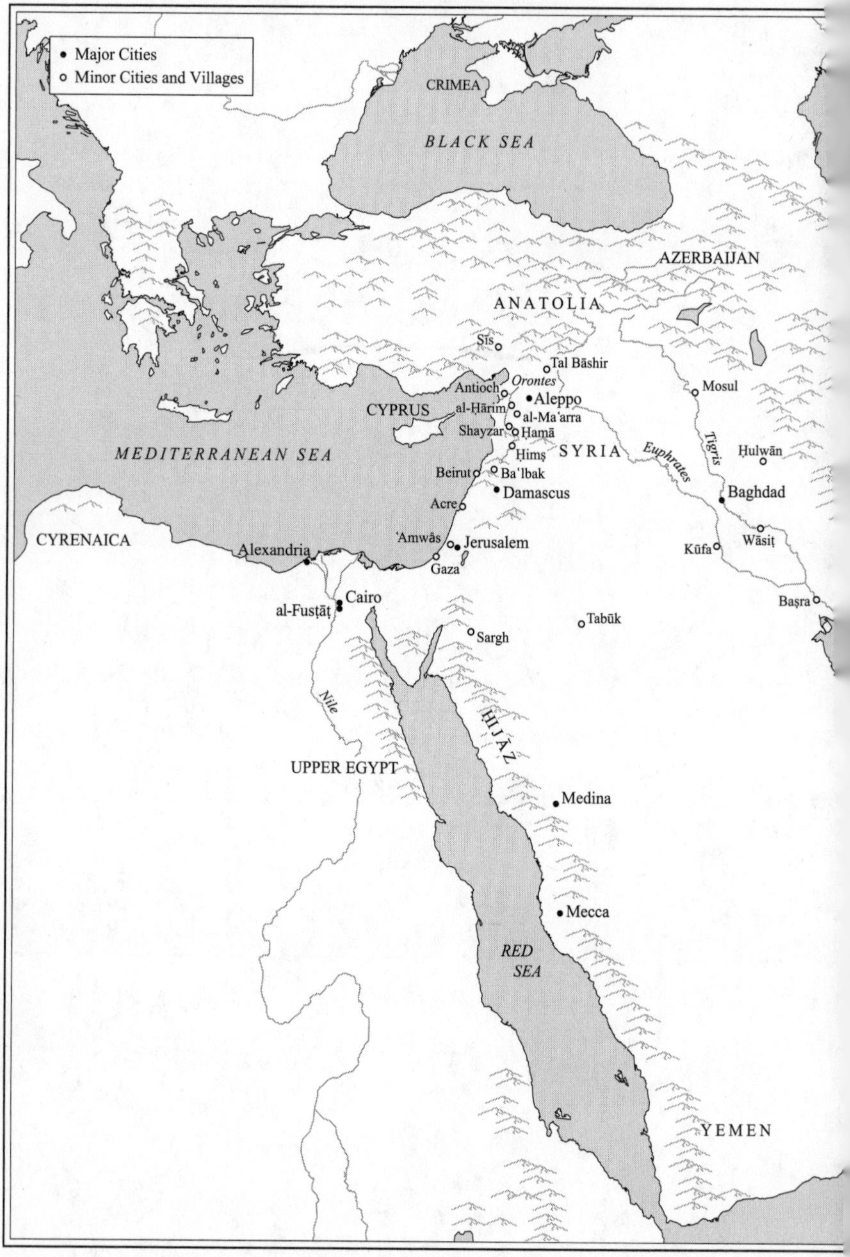

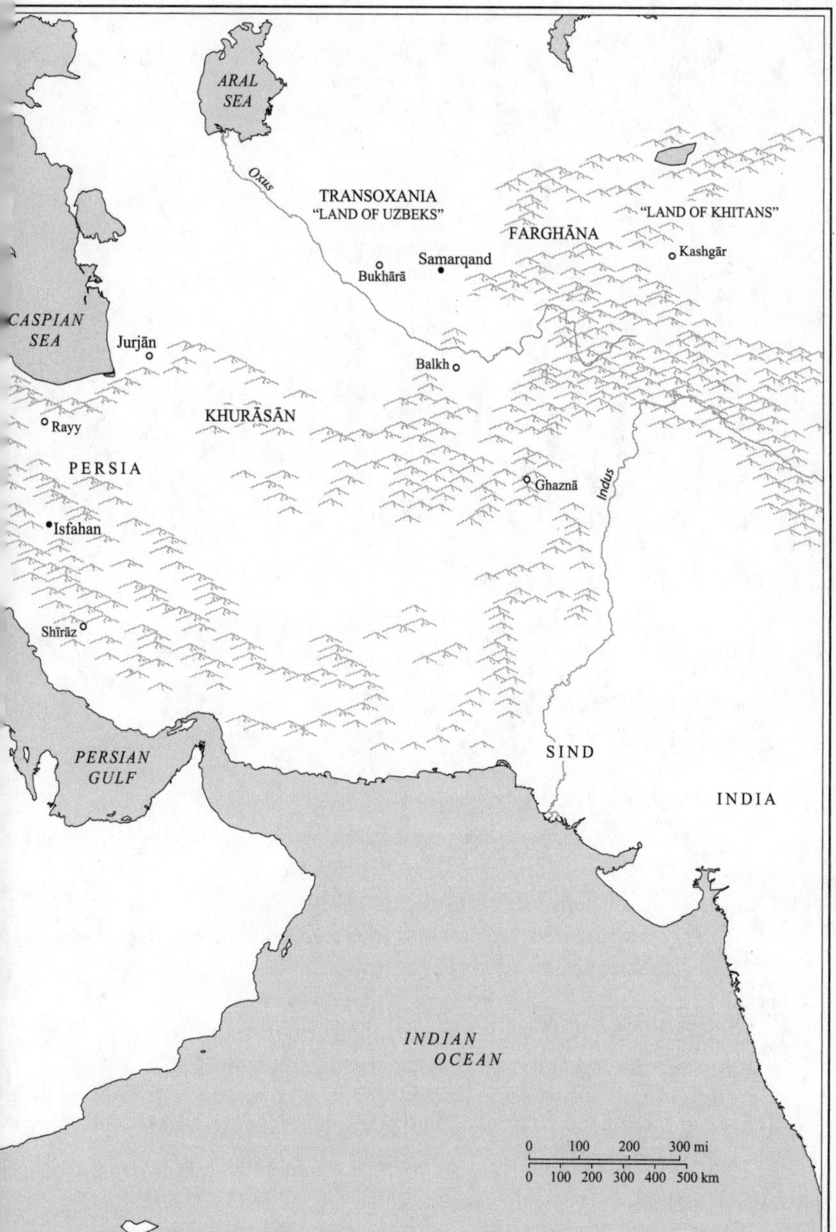
ARAL SEA
Oxus
TRANSOXANIA
"LAND OF UZBEKS"
"LAND OF KHITANS"
FARGHĀNA
Kashgār
Samarqand
Bukhārā
CASPIAN SEA
Jurjān
Balkh
KHURĀSĀN
Rayy
PERSIA
Ghaznā
Indus
Isfahan
Shīrāz
PERSIAN GULF
SIND
INDIA
INDIAN OCEAN
0 100 200 300 mi
0 100 200 300 400 500 km

Merits of the Plague

Preface of the Author

My Lord, facilitate this for me and help me. All praise is due to God in all affairs, and we seek refuge in Him from the plight of the damned. We ask Him, the Pardoner and Forgiver, for forgiveness and pardon in this life and the next. We bear witness that there is no god but God—none share His Divinity. He is the Determiner of provisions and life spans. He closes the gap for those who fall short in worshipping Him by way of His Grace, a Grace that never falls short. We bear witness that Muhammad is His servant and Messenger, the pure and chosen one, creation's fortress against terrible afflictions. Muhammad will be the advocate for those who are humiliated by grievous sin on the Day of Judgment, and Muhammad's intercession will be accepted by God because he is free from the wrath of the Mighty King. May God everlastingly bless, send prayers to, and bestow peace on him and his righteous and God-fearing family, during the darkness of night and the lightness of day.

When my colleagues, may God benefit them, repeatedly asked me to collect all reports on the plague, comment on the unusual ones, facilitate an understanding of them, interpret them, clarify their implications for the religious law, and give an account of their types, I acquiesced to their desire. I ask God for aid in all endeavors.

I organized this book in five chapters: on the plague's origin; on the plague's definition; on the proof of the plague being an opportunity for martyrdom; on the religious laws regulating the leaving or entering of a land in which the plague strikes; and on what the religious law says one should do after the plague occurs.[1]

I titled this book *Offering Aid on the Merits of the Plague*.

I ask that God not make the results of my work something evil—and I ask that He, the Exalted and Glorious, through His grace and generosity, bless its culmination with excellence!

CHAPTER ONE

ORIGINS OF THE PLAGUE

I.1

Hadiths That Prove That the Plague Is a Divine Punishment

Al-Bukhārī and Muslim recorded that Usāma ibn Zayd said that God's Messenger said:

> "This suffering is an abomination and a punishment by which people before you were punished."[1]

Ibn Abī Shayba records that the Prophet said:

> "This plague is a punishment, the remnant of the punishment by which people before you were punished . . ."[2]

In one version found in ʿAbd al-Razzāq's *Collection*, God's Messenger said:

> "This pestilence is a punishment by which God destroyed some peoples. Some of it has lingered upon the earth, and it comes and goes from time to time."[3]

Al-Ṭabarānī records that the Prophet said:

> "This ailment—or illness—is a punishment, by which some peoples who came before you were punished, but which persisted afterward upon the earth. It goes away for a time and returns for a time."[4]

Al-Ṭabarānī also records the following version:

> ʿAbd al-Raḥmān ibn ʿAwf informed them, while he was on the road to Syria when the plague had struck it, that the

Prophet said: "This ailment or illness is a punishment, by which those before you were punished."[5]

HADITHS THAT PROVE THE PLAGUE IS A PUNISHMENT AND A MERCY

Imām Aḥmad said, citing Abū ʿAsīb, that God's Messenger said:

> "The Angel Gabriel came offering me pestilential fever and plague. I took the fever for Medina and sent the plague to Syria, because the plague is a martyrdom and mercy for my community and a punishment for the disbelievers."[6]

Anas ibn Mālik's hadith, recorded by Ibn Abī al-Dunya, comes close to explaining the hadith above. In this hadith, when he and another man went to ʿĀʾisha, the other man asked:

> "Mother of the believers! Would you teach us about the great earthquake?"
>
> She said: "When people seek to make fornication permissible, drink wine and play lutes and tambourines, God in His heavens becomes angry and commands the earth: 'Quake under them! But, if they repent and refrain, cease.' If they do not, He rents the land beneath them."
>
> "Mother of the believers! Is it a punishment for them?"
>
> "Not exactly. It is a reminder and a mercy for the believers, but a punishment and a display of wrath for the disbelievers."
>
> Anas said: "No other hadith that I heard brought me as much joy as this one."

HADITHS THAT CLARIFY THE PUNISHMENT AND UPON WHOM IT IS SENT

ʿAlī ibn Abī Ṭālib said:

> There once was a prophet whose people disobeyed him.
>
> A voice called out to him: "Shall we wipe them out with famine?"
>
> He replied, "No."
>
> The voice then asked: "Shall we give one of their enemies power over them?"
>
> "No," said the prophet, "but whatever you do should be a vile form of death."
>
> So it was that God subjected them to the plague. He made it decimate their population and burn their hearts . . .[7]

The isnad of this hadith is acceptable.[8] After discovering the hadith above, I located a report with the rationale for David's building of the holy temple in Ibn Isḥāq's work *The Origin*:

> God revealed to David that the children of Israel had increased in their disobedience to God. Therefore, God gave them a choice between three Divine punishments: that they be struck with drought for two years; that their enemies subjugate them for two months; or that God sends them the plague for three days.
>
> David presented the choice to them. They said: "You are our prophet, choose for us."
>
> He said: "Famine is a disgraceful trial, which would be unbearable. And if we were subjugated to our enemies, nothing would remain afterward." So he chose the plague for them.
>
> By the time the sun had set, seventy thousand had died—some say one hundred thousand. So David implored God for relief, and God lifted the plague from them.
>
> David said: "God, the Exalted, has shown you mercy, so give thanks to God for the amount that he tested you!" He

then began building the temple, which his son, Solomon, completed—peace be upon both of them.[9]

Abū Jaʿfar al-Ṭabarī recorded this from Saʿīd ibn Jubayr:

> Moses commanded his people from among the children of Israel to wipe ram's blood on the doors. This happened after the five divine signs came to the Pharaoh's people—the flood and other things God mentions in the verse: "and we sent against them the flood, the locusts . . ."[10]
>
> When the Egyptians still did not believe nor release the children of Israel to Moses, he ordered his people: "Let each man slaughter a ram, dip his palm into its blood, and wipe it on his door."
>
> When they did this, an Egyptian asked the Israelites: "Why have you put blood on your doors?"
>
> They said: "The Exalted God will deliver upon you a punishment that will kill you, and you will thereby be destroyed."
>
> The Egyptian then asked: "Will God only know you through this sign?"
>
> They said: "This is what our prophet commanded."
>
> When they woke up the next day, seventy thousand of Pharaoh's people had been pierced by the plague. They were still burying their dead when evening came.
>
> With that, Pharaoh asked Moses:
>
> "Pray to your Lord for us by virtue of the promise He has made to you. If you remove this punishment from us, we will surely believe in you and let the Children of Israel go with you."[11]
>
> So Moses prayed to his Lord, and God lifted the plague upon them.[12]

This hadith is attributed to one of the Companions with a strong isnad.[13]

The upshot of this is that those afflicted by the plague in Usāma ibn Zayd's hadith are Pharaoh's people. Qāḍī ʿIyāḍ thought that it was rather "a punishment for the Israelites," and that some said that the number of Israelites who died in a single hour was twenty thousand—others said seventy thousand. In my opinion, the second number is the correct one, but they were Pharaoh's people who died from the plague and not the Israelites.

I came across a well-sourced account for this claim, which al-Ṭabarī quotes from Sayyār:

> There was a man named Balaam, who was one of those whose prayers were answered by God.* Around this time Moses had joined the Israelites, and he desired the land of Canaan that Balaam occupied, so the Canaanites were terrified of Moses.
>
> The Canaanites went to find Balaam and said: "Pray to God against the Israelites!"
>
> Balaam said: "Not until I consult with my Lord."
>
> Then Balaam consulted with Him. A voice said to Balaam, "Do not pray against them—they are my servants, and their prophet is with them."
>
> The Canaanites gave Balaam a gift, and he received it. Then they returned with the request that he pray against Moses and the Israelites. Again, he said, "Not until I consult my Lord."
>
> Balaam consulted again with God and, this time, received no response.
>
> Then the Canaanites said: "If your Lord did not want you to pray against them, He would have forbidden it, just like He did the first time."
>
> So he began to pray against them, but the prayer that flowed off his tongue was against his own people, even though he desired to pray for them. Instead, he prayed that God give victory to Moses and his army. So the Canaanites cursed him.
>
> Balaam said: "No words are coming out of my mouth but these! However, I will offer you a suggestion in the hopes that it may lead to their destruction. God abhors fornication, and

*Balaam is a figure mentioned in the Hebrew Bible. Compare this account with Numbers 22 and Numbers 31:16.

> if the Israelites engage in it, they will be wiped out. So send the women out. The Israelites may take them in, because they are travelers. Then they might fornicate with them and thereby ensure their own destruction." The Canaanites did exactly that.
>
> The king of the Canaanites had a daughter who had the kind of beauty of which only God knows. Her father told her not to give herself to anyone but Moses so that the Israelites might succumb to fornication. But the head of one of the Israelites' tribes wanted her despite her objections. "I will only give myself to Moses," she protested.
>
> "I am close to Moses . . . ," he insisted. She sent a message to her father, and he gave her permission, and she gave herself to him.
>
> A man from Aaron's clan approached the two of them with a spear and pierced them both. God gave this man from Aaron's clan enormous strength, and he fixed the two of them on his spear and then lifted them both for the people to see. Thus, God subjected the Israelites to the plague, and seventy thousand of them died.[14]

Al-Ṭabarī has a simpler version of the story above. In that version, he states that after Balaam's prayers went unanswered, he offered the following advice:

> "The only option that remains is trickery and ploy. Beautify the women, give them wares to sell, and send them to the Israelite encampment, so that even if just one of them dabbled in fornication, you would be done with them." The Canaanites did exactly that.
>
> When the women entered the encampment, a Canaanite whose name was Cozbi daughter of Zur sauntered past an Israelite leader, Zimri son of Salu, who was the chief of the tribe of Simeon. He approached her and took her hand, enchanted by her beauty. He was entranced with her, even though he was standing in front of Moses, may peace and blessings be upon him.

> Zimri said to Moses: "I know what you are going to say—'this woman is forbidden to you.'"
>
> Moses said: "Correct. She is forbidden to you. Do not go near her."
>
> Zimri said: "By God, I cannot obey you in this." Then he entered his tent with her and lay with her.
>
> Then God sent the plague upon the Israelites. Phinehas the son of Eleazar, the son of Aaron was Moses's representative, and he was blessed with great moral integrity and strength in the ability to strike with violence. He had been away. When the plague came and ravaged the Israelites, he was given the news. He grabbed his lance and then entered Zimri's tent. He fixed them both upon his lance while they were in the act of copulation.
>
> Then he went out with the two of them and began to say: "O God, this is what we do to those who disobey You!" And the plague was lifted.
>
> The estimated number that perished from the plague between the time Zimri lay with the woman until the time he was killed was seventy thousand.

At a minimum, al-Ṭabarī says, the number was twenty thousand. Al-Ṭabarī recorded this story, which I have summarized, in many different versions. But only these two accounts above mention the plague. The narrators of both are trustworthy and each of the versions strengthens the other.

Another report has God sending the plague against a faction of the Israelites, the ones referenced in the Qur'an: "Those who fled their homes, fearing death, by the thousands . . ."[15] The explanation of this will be discussed later in the book, as well as the view of the one who claimed that they went out fleeing from the plague.

The well-known judge Qāḍī ʿIyāḍ holds that there are two ways of reading the hadith. The first is that it documents this as the first time the plague occurred in the land; that the plague struck people—these Israelites specifically. The second is that it shows that they were punished by the plague.

I see no contradiction between these two readings. It is possible to read it as saying that it was the earliest punishment of its kind that struck them. One may then reconcile the two readings by supposing that the plague had previously struck a people other than them, but not as a punishment, and then it struck them for the first time as a punishment. Thus, the fact that they were the first is qualified by the fact that they were the first punished by it, not that they were the first to experience the plague. But it is plain to see that this latter way of reconciling the two readings is unlikely to be correct, since the plague punishes the body beyond any shadow of a doubt, regardless of whether its purpose is mercy or not.

CHAPTER TWO

UNDERSTANDING THE PLAGUE

2.1

Defining the Plague

THE ETYMOLOGY OF THE ARABIC TERM FOR PLAGUE

The word for "plague" in Arabic, according to al-Jawharī, is etymologically derived from the root verb ṭa-ʿa-na, which means to pierce or stab. People altered the meaning from this root and made the plague something that signifies widespread death, like a pestilence. It is said that when the plague strikes someone, "he is pierced," just as if they were stabbed by a spear.

THE PLAGUE'S CHARACTERISTICS AND CAUSES

Ibrahīm al-Ḥarbī said:

> A pestilence can be defined as a plague and any widespread epidemic. . . . The plague is well known; it consists of the pustules by which God tries whom He wills. . . .[1]

Ibn al-ʿArabī said:

> "The pierced" are those struck by the plague. The plague is an overpowering ailment that chokes out breath similar to al-dhubḥa, a throat disease.* It is called "the plague" on account of the prevalence of its affliction and the speed with which it kills, so anything like it is classified as such.[2]

*Although, in modern times, al-dhubḥa is associated with diphtheria or angina, in Ibn Ḥajar's time, al-dhubḥa was a term of art that described a life-threatening disease of the throat, sometimes obstructing the breath with an ulceration behind the tongue.

Abū al-Walīd al-Bājī said:

> The plague is an ailment that spreads to many people from every direction, in contrast to the typical illnesses that afflict people. The ailment of those afflicted by the plague is one and the same, in contrast to other moments in time in which people suffer from different diseases.[3]

Ibn al-Tīn cited al-Dāwūdī, who said:

> The plague consists of a swelling that erupts in the soft flesh of the body and in every crease. The correct understanding is that a plague is a pestilence.[4]

Ibn al-Athīr said in *The End*:

> The Prophet said: "The end of my community will be by the sword and the plague." By "the sword," he meant death by an enemy's spears, and by "the plague" he meant the widespread sickness and pestilence that corrupts the air, which, in turn, corrupts the temperaments and the body. The aim of the hadith is to assert that the destruction of the Muslim community will happen mostly through civil strife, which involves the shedding of blood, and through a pestilence. The term "plague" is repeated in many hadiths.[5]

After mentioning the hadith above, Ibn ʿAbd al-Barr said:

> The plague is a lump, like those that erupt during the ghudda disease that can be found in camels.* The lumps erupt on the armpits and the lower abdomen.

---

*Ghudda was "a deadly disease of camels characterized by swellings similar to those of bubonic plague" and would have been well-known to audiences of these reports. Lawrence Conrad, "*Tāʿūn* and *Wabāʾ*: Conceptions of Plague and Pestilence in Early Islam," *Journal of the Economic and Social History of the Orient,* 25/3 (1982): 298.

A different expert said, "It erupts on the hands and fingers and elsewhere on the body, as God wills it." According to Qāḍī 'Iyāḍ:

> The term "plague," at its core, is defined by the sores that erupt on the body. Meanwhile, the term "pestilence," which comprises the totality of all such diseases, is called a "plague" by virtue of the death that occurs from it. Every plague is a pestilence, but not every pestilence is a plague. Abū Mūsā's hadith is evidence of this: "The plague is the piercing caused by your enemies among the jinn." The pestilence in Syria that occurs in many reports was, in fact, the plague—the 'Amwās plague—and it manifested as sores.

Al-Nawawī summed up Qāḍī 'Iyāḍ's point in his *Commentary on Muslim's Authentic Hadith*:

> The plague is a well-known disease. It consists of intensely painful pustules and swellings, which erupt on the body. Their eruption is accompanied by a fiery inflammation; the surrounding area then blackens, and darkens or reddens into a dingy purple. Other symptoms include heart palpitations and vomiting. The pustules usually appear near the groin or the armpits as well as the hands, fingers, and the rest of the body."[6]

In a different work of his, *The Garden*, al-Nawawī added:

> Some explained the plague as resulting from the flowing of blood to a body part. Most of them thought that plague is the stirring up of blood and its puffing up.

Al-Mutawallī said:

> The plague is similar to leprosy. The body parts of whoever it strikes deteriorate, and his flesh falls off.[7]

Al-Ghazālī said in *The Primer*:

> The plague swells the entire body with blood and is accompanied by fever; or blood flows to the extremities, swelling and reddening those places and destroying the body part if its condition is not immediately rectified.[8]

Avicenna and other medical experts said:

> The plague is a poisonous substance that produces deadly swellings. The swelling occurs in the soft, glandular parts of the body, usually under the armpits or behind the ears or the groin. . . .
>
> The cause of the swellings is bad blood predisposed to spoiling and corruption. It transforms into a poisonous substance that corrupts the body part and the surrounding area, and conveys a corrosive quality to the heart, which then produces vomiting, nausea, fainting, and heart palpitations. The swellings in the soft glandular parts of the body are due to the blood's corruption, as the bad blood is only taken up by those parts of the body that are weak by nature. The worst of the corrupted blood is that which is taken up by those soft glandular parts from the chief organs. The black plague bubo is the most dangerous of the plague swellings, while the least is the red and then the yellow. . . .
>
> Incidences of plague increase in times of pestilence, and in pestilential places. For this reason, the term "pestilence" is applied to plagues and vice versa. . . .
>
> The pestilence is a corruption of the substance of air, which is the material for the generation of the spirit and its source of sustenance. For that reason, the life of a person—nay, the life of all creatures!—is impossible without breathing, such that, when animals are deprived of breathing air, they die.

To sum up what we have gathered from the preceding discussion, the plague is of many types:

The most well-known type of plague is the one in which swellings erupt on the body, especially in the soft, glandular flesh.* Sometimes it occurs on hands, fingers, and all parts of the body, but the latter is rare when compared to those that occur in the soft, glandular flesh.

A second type of plague can also occur in any part of the body as sores and pustules, but especially in the body's soft, glandular flesh, as opposed to other areas.

A third type of plague is what chokes out the breath of life similar to al-dhubḥa, the throat disease. But al-dhubḥa is not plague in itself; rather, it is included as a type of plague due to the way it may resemble it. For that reason, the condition of one who is afflicted by it varies depending on whether it is at a time of plague or not. I say this only because an authentic hadith has established—as will be explained in the coming chapter—that "the plague will never enter Medina." At the same time, another authentic hadith has established that the Prophet treated his Companion Asʿad ibn Zurāra's throat disease (al-dhubḥa) with cautery. The same is true of al-Barāʾ ibn Maʿrūr who were both in Medina. It may be the case that the Prophet's treatment was before he prayed to God, asking that the plague not enter Medina.

A fourth type of plague strikes a body part and causes it to deteriorate, just as in leprosy, as al-Mutawallī discussed earlier. I have seen an example of this in the earliest generation of Muslims: "Ziyād wrote Muʿāwiya and mentioned the following in the context of a story: 'A plague bubo appeared on his finger, and he did not live to see another Friday.'"[9] The report notes that his finger deteriorated, and they advised him to amputate it lest the deterioration spread. He did not do that, and he died.

---

*Avicenna identifies three specific areas of the body as sites for buboes: the armpit, the groin, and behind the ears, which he calls the three maghābin. What unites them is their soft and glandular character. See Nahyan Fancy and Monica Green, "Plague and the Fall of Baghdad (1258)" in *Medical History*, 65/2, 167n52.

HEAVENLY CAUSES AND EARTHLY CAUSES OF THE PLAGUE

According to ʿAlāʾ al-Dīn ibn al-Nafīs in his *Concise Book of Medicine*, the pestilence begins with the corruption that occurs in the air's substance due to celestial and terrestrial causes. He identifies the following as the terrestrial causes: brackish water; piles of corpses, as can occur during a battle when the dead are left unburied; mucky ground; and masses of rotting matter, along with an increase in the number of insects and frogs. The celestial causes for the plague are an abundance of meteors and shooting stars at the end of summer and in the fall; an increase in southerly and easterly winds during December and January; as well as numerous signs pointing to rain during the winter, but without it raining. All of that is based on observable experience. Al-Jāḥiẓ remarked that when the magpie senses such winds, it flees from that land. Similarly, rats flee their underground burrows.

2.2

Plague Is Not Synonymous with Pestilence

The following hadiths offer evidence that the plague and pestilence are not synonyms—rather, the plague is a type of pestilence.*

Abū Hurayra said that God's Messenger said:

*In English, "the plague" refers to both the universal term for epidemics but also to the specific illness caused by *Yersinia pestis* that is the subject of this book. We have sought to distinguish between plague and pestilence here to approximate the distinction in Arabic between ṭaʿūn (the plague in its bubonic, pneumonic, and septicemic forms) and wabāʾ (pestilence, plague, epidemic).

> "There are angels on the mountain paths on the way to Medina—neither the plague nor the Antichrist* will enter it."[10]

In Anas's rendition, God's Messenger said:

> "The Antichrist will come to Medina but find angels guarding its gates, and so will not enter it, nor will the plague, unless God wills, may He be exalted."[11]

ʿĀʾisha said:

> "We went to Medina when it was the most pestilential of God's earth, may God be exalted."[12]

On this issue, there is also Bilāl's statement:

> "O God, curse Shayba ibn Rabīʿa, ʿUtba ibn Rabīʿa, and Umayya ibn Khalaf, as they have driven us from our land to a land of pestilence."

If the plague was the same thing as the pestilence, these two hadiths would contradict each other. But there is no contradiction because the plague is a certain type of pestilence.[13] When ʿĀʾisha used the phrase "most pestilential" to describe Medina, she merely meant that there was an abundance of fevers there.

Abū ʿAsīb's aforementioned hadith is evidence that when God offered him a choice between plague and fever, the Prophet selected fever over the plague and accepted that fever would come to Medina. Then he prayed to God, and God relocated it to al-Juḥfa, as has been established in both al-Bukhārī and Muslim's *Authentic Hadith* on the authority of ʿĀʾisha. But pockets of the fever lingered in Medina. This is clear in the story of the ʿUraynī people in Anas's hadith, recorded in al-Bukhārī

---

*The Dajjāl, or "Great Deceiver," is often translated as the "Antichrist"—one prophesied to emerge in the last days to beguile people, in part with claims of his own godship.

and Muslim's *Authentic Hadith*, that the people of ʿUrayna "found Medina unhealthy for them"; one version said, "This land is pestilential." In another narration, it is said that "their bodies became ill, and the color of their skin turned yellow."

The two hadiths can be reconciled in the following way: The fever struck those people of Medina who resided there and whoever arrived there from the outside. When the Prophet called upon God to send the fever from them to al-Juḥfa, God lifted it from the people of Medina, save a few rare exceptions; those who did not comport with Medina's weather, for instance, got ill from it.

Still, the pestilence brought about a great death during the time of ʿUmar. Abū al-Aswad al-Duʾalī's report states: "I came to Medina, and it had been struck by an illness. The people were rapidly dying in great numbers, so I sat with ʿUmar. . . ."[14]

This hadith does not contradict the fact that the Prophet called for God to lift the pestilence from Medina, because it rarely occurred there. As for the plague, there is no report that it occurred there, from the time of the Prophet to our time, God be praised. God willing, in the third chapter I will discuss the wisdom of the fact that the plague never enters Medina, even though it has also been established that its occurrence is a martyrdom.

What is clear from the preceding discussion is that the plague is more limited in its meaning than the pestilence. The reports we discussed earlier that mentioned the plague as pestilence do not necessarily mean that every pestilence is a plague, but rather indicate the opposite: that every plague is a pestilence. Since the pestilence results in great mortality, as the plague does too, the term "pestilence" is used to refer to it.

The plague is a distinct type of pestilence because of its cause, the equivalent of which does not exist in any of the other pestilences. It is caused by "the pricks of the jinn." In my view, this fact does not conflict with the opinion of the physicians, discussed previously, that the plague results from poisonous matter or a stirring up of blood or the flowing of it to a body part, and so on. This is because there is nothing that prevents these from being ultimately generated by a hidden act of a jinn's piercing. The piercing can generate poisonous matter, or cause the blood to stir up or flow toward a body part. Physicians cannot object to the claim that the plague is caused by the jinn's piercing because the pricks of the jinn cannot be grasped by reason or sensory experience; rather, we can only attain knowledge of it from the report of the Law Giver. Physicians may only speak of what results from that piercing to the degree permitted by the principles of their science.[15] But God knows best.

Indeed, the explanation that the plague is caused by the pricks of the jinn resolves the problems that otherwise are present in the explanation of physicians and others who claim that plague is caused by the corruption of air. Ibn al-Qayyim discussed this in *The Gift* and refuted the corruption of air explanation in the following ways:

First, Ibn al-Qayyim asserted that it occurs during the most balanced seasons and in regions with the healthiest air and the most pleasant water. He added that if plague were caused by foul air, it would afflict all people and animals. But we find many people and animals plague-stricken, even as those belonging to the same species with similar temperaments right next to them are not afflicted with plague. The plague has been seen taking the lives of all the people of a certain house in a certain region while not entering at all the house next to it. Or plague enters a home but only afflicts some of its inhabitants. It has also been observed that the plague was sometimes lighter during times in which the air was corrupted than when the air was healthy.

Ibn al-Qayyim further added that the air's corruption necessarily causes changes in the humors and thereby an increase in diseases and illnesses. Yet the plague kills without there being other diseases, or with there being mild diseases. Furthermore, he added that if it were caused by the air's corruption, it would spread to the entire body through its continuous inhalation. But the plague bubo only occurs in a specific part of the body and does not extend beyond that, and it usually kills the person whose body part was affected.

Ibn al-Qayyim also argued that if the plague were the result of corrupt air, it would persist at all times on the earth, because the air is healthy sometimes and corrupt other times. But the plague comes without any observable or logical pattern. It arrives one year, and then is absent for several years.

Lastly, Ibn al-Qayyim said that each illness that results from natural causes can be treated using natural remedies, as established in the sound hadith: "God did not send down an illness without sending down a cure; knowledge of the cure is from knowledge of the illness; ignorance of the cure is from ignorance of the illness."[16] But this plague has thwarted the physicians' treatments. The most proficient masters of medicine have accepted that there is no cure for it at all, and that there is no defense against it except through the One who created it and decreed its course. But God knows best.

In *The Meaning of the Reports*, al-Kalābādhī says the following:

> Ailments and pestilences are each a disease like the rest of the diseases that afflict people due to their natures and the overpowering of one or more of the humors even if they are not caused by the piercing of a human or a jinn.
>
> Thus, it is possible to classify plague in two ways. The first is a disease that is not caused by the jinn: an ailment or pestilence that occurs due to the preponderance of some humors, be it blood or yellow bile, when it is burned or not.[17] The second is as something caused by the jinn's pricking. This can be like the sore that results in illness or an ailment that afflicts a person from the burning of blood and its overpowering of the humors, resulting in the tearing of skin and exposing of the flesh, even though one has not been visibly pierced there.
>
> To this also belongs the piercing of a human, as God, the Exalted, says: "If a q-r-ḥ afflicts you, a similar q-r-ḥ afflicted others."[18] The word "q-r-ḥ" can take the form "qarḥun" in some Qur'anic recitations, and "qurḥun" in others. The qarḥun pronunciation means laceration. The qurḥun form means an abscess. Just as the piercings and abscesses are also called sores, the Prophet and his Companions called

> the plague an ailment or illness. God, the Exalted, has said: "If you have been caused pain, then they are in pain just as you are."[19] Pain means ailment, and ailment refers to disease and illness. Just as one of the two forms of reading q-r-ḥ—that is, as laceration or abscess—do not negate the other's meaning, likewise the two hadiths do not negate one another, as plague can be read either as the result of a jinn's prick or as a pestilence. Just as it is possible for q-r-ḥ to mean both laceration and sore, likewise it is possible for the plague to be the pricking of jinn or an illness.[20]

The gist of his discussion is that calling the plague "a pestilence" or "an ailment" or "an illness" is construed as meaning something other than its being "the pricks of the jinn." What is apparent from what he has mentioned is that this is not the only way of looking at things. The term "pestilence" applies to anything that causes much death, as was discussed, and it is broader in meaning than the term "plague." As for the terms "illness" and "ailment," each one applies to every disease, either the plague or something else.

The fact that some ailments occur in the plague due to the overpowering of natures does not prevent plague from being caused by the piercing of the jinn. It is possible that the jinn's piercing results in those physical changes that agitate the plague-stricken body, boiling the blood, which makes the blood attain a foul quality that physicians misidentify as the true cause of plague, according to the stipulations of the fundamental principles of their science. However, that does not disqualify the jinn from being the true first cause. But God knows best.

2.3
"The Plague Is the Pricks of the Jinn"

The following hadiths offer context for the debate surrounding the hadith that contains the phrase "the plague is the pricks of the jinn."

The Messenger of God said:

> "The end of my community will be by the sword and the plague."
>
> "Oh, Messenger of God," it was said to him, "we understand what the sword is, but what is the plague?"
>
> "The pricks of your enemies among the jinn, and there is a martyrdom for each who dies of them."[21]

"THE END OF MY COMMUNITY WILL BE BY THE SWORD AND THE PLAGUE"

The apparent meaning of the hadith—and God knows best—is that it is a request to God, because in one of the isnads from the Companion Abū Mūsā, the text says so explicitly: "Oh Lord, make the end of my community by an ailment."[22] In another narration from Abū Mūsā al-Ashaʿrī's brother, God's Messenger said: "Oh Lord, make the end of my community in such a way that they are killed in Your path by the sword and the plague." Our Shaykh Abū al-Faḍl ibn al-Ḥusayn recited the following poem on the meaning of the hadith above, during the lecture recitation of his hadith collection:

> Honor the umma with goodness, Oh Lord!
> An umma You brought to this world and what's after!
> An umma martyred by sword and by plague,
> pricked by their foes among the jinn.

One of our older contemporaries held the opposite position. He noted that the well-preserved version—"the end of my community will be by the sword and the plague"—is a description of the state of affairs rather than a prayer to God. Ibn al-Athīr, in *The End*, wrote:

> The Prophet meant that the end of the community will be largely through the civil strife that results in a great shedding of blood—and also by the pestilence.

We should reject Ibn al-Athīr's claim that the hadith's phrasing as a prayer is not well preserved on account of the authenticated hadiths I cited earlier. As I will discuss in the coming pages, the text of Abū Bakr al-Ṣiddīq's prayer testifies to that.

2.4
A Response to the Objections to the Hadith

"THE END OF MY COMMUNITY WILL BE BY THE SWORD AND THE PLAGUE"

The following offers a response to those who impugn the hadith "the end of my community will be by the sword and the plague," by citing the fact that most people died of something other than the sword and the plague. They add that had the hadith been true, everyone would have died from one or the other.

In the prophetic hadith that "the end of my community will be by the sword and the plague," according to Ibn al-Athīr, the Prophet meant that most of the destruction of his community will be by the civil strife in which blood is shed as well as the pestilence. He did not consider the hadith cited above with the phrase "the end . . ." to be a supplication to God. I have already proposed that it is possible to construe the first version of this hadith as a supplication, even though it was phrased as a description. It is possible that the Prophet prayed to God on behalf of his community using general terms, but that God answered his prayers for only some members of his community. In this way, the general term "community" actually denoted a particular group among Muslims—but not all of them. It is also possible that the Prophet intended the phrase "my community" to be a shorthand for his Companions or a group that possessed a specific quality, such as the few who were the most righteous of his community. In this way, the general term "community" indicates something specific.

Concerning the first group—the Companions—the objection is raised that the Companions did not all die due to one or both reasons. The same objection is raised with the notion that only "the best" of his community died of the civil strife and the pestilence because most of them died of something else. Another case is closely related to problems related to the interpretation of the term "my community" as denoting the Companions: The Prophet prayed to God for the forgiveness of the believers. Yet, for Sunnis at least, definitive evidence establishes that a group of them will be punished in hell and then subsequently extricated because of the Prophet's intercession.

A contrast to the case above is shown in the Prophet's supplication to God, imploring Him that He not destroy the Prophet's community by a famine, or floods, or confound them with partisanship. The Prophet was given the first two and denied the remaining. In the middle of another hadith, the Prophet states:

> "I asked my Lord not to destroy my community by a famine, nor to put their enemies in positions of power over them, nor to allow partisanship arise among them, such that they come to harm each other. So He said to me: 'Muhammad! When I execute a judgment, it cannot be overcome. For your community I grant that I will not destroy them by a famine, and I will not put their enemies in posi-

tions of power over them, to the point of plundering the heart of their lands . . . unless they begin to tear each other apart.'"[23]

In another hadith, the Prophet said:

"I prayed to God to relieve my community of four things. He relieved them of two, and he refused to relieve them of two. I called upon God to relieve them of being pelted by stones from the sky, being swallowed by the earth, confounding them with partisanship, and having some of them sow violence on others. So God relieved them of the earthquakes and the stones, and refused to relieve them of the other two."[24]

Another example is what the Companion Jābir said:

When this verse from the Qur'an was sent down—"Say: He is capable of sending upon you punishment from above . . ."[25] the Prophet of God interjected: "I seek protection in your countenance!"

". . . or from below your feet . . ." the Prophet again interjected, "I seek protection in your countenance!"

". . . or confound you with partisanship and cause some of you to sow violence on others." The Messenger of God said: "These two are the easier among these torments."[26]

Yet, a part of the Muslim community, in some lands, has been struck by stones from the sky, earthquakes, and floods, and has suffered conquest by unbelieving enemies. This fact indicates that the hadith's negation of these occurrences is merely a negation of them striking the totality of Muslims. The occurrence of these hardships to some of them does not detract from the soundness of the hadith, on account of the fact that "my community" can validly convey in its meaning both "all" and "part."

The same can be said with respect to the hadith we are discussing in this chapter, "The end of my community will be by the sword and the plague." The term "my community" is capable of conveying the intention to denote all of the community or a part of it. What subsequently happened in the community's history showed that the phrase denotes just part of it; just as what subsequently happened shows that the term in the hadith on famine and partisanship denotes all of it. However, it does not refer to "all" in the sense of the entirety of the community from beginning to end, such that all who have accepted the Prophet's call die off and the only ones remaining are those given the opportunity to follow him. Rather, it refers to all who are present in a particular age, in all of the lands belonging to the Muhammadan community. The dying off of all believers will only happen after the occurrence of miraculous signs of the end of time. This is when Jesus son of Mary will die following his return, those who truly believe in the one God will die, and no one will remain on the face of the earth who says, "There is no god but God," for the final hour is upon them. This has been established in an authenticated hadith. Concerning what occurs before that final hour, the learned scholars disagree on certain questions—such as, "Will the earth be absent of anyone to undertake the hajj for God's sake?"—but this is not the place to discuss this issue.

One of the latter-day scholars alleges that the intended meaning of the hadith on "the sword and the plague" is the destruction of the community at the end of time, and the "piercing" explains the chaos before the final judgment mentioned in the other hadith, because the latter contains the term "killing." Meanwhile, the term for the plague refers to the wind that will take the souls of the believers at the end of time. Yet, one variant of the hadith on "the sword and the plague" contains the phrase "it takes them in their armpits." In this way, it is plain to see that the interpretation of it as referring to events before the final judgment is strained and unlikely to be the case. If I did not fear that people would be duped by it, I would not have introduced it as an aside to warn them away from it.

Whoever considers the full context of the hadiths that we

will discuss in the next chapter knows the inadequacy of what this latter-day scholar alleged. All that is needed to rebut it is the consensus of the religious scholars that death by the plague is meritorious, whereas his position requires that death by plague has no merit in it and that the hadith on the plague is merely a description of what will happen at the end times.

Abū al-ʿAbbās al-Qurṭubī argues that the meaning of "community" in the phrase "the end of my community" refers to the Companions. Al-Qurṭubī notes:

> The intention behind Muʿādh's hadith saying that the plague is "the supplication of your Prophet" is that the Prophet called upon God to obliterate his community "by the sword and the plague." One narration from Abū Qilāba has the word "and" between "the sword" and "the plague." But one of our scholars has said, "The authentic phrasing is 'the sword *or* the plague'—that is, one of those two hardships. This means that both would not afflict them at the same time. . . ."

Al-Qurṭubī continued:

> "It seems to me that two narrations are authentic in terms of their meaning. The elucidation of that meaning is that the Prophet's intent in employing the term "community" in the hadith is only for his Companions, which relies on the fact that his prayer was fulfilled when he prayed to God on behalf of his community that God not empower their external enemies over them; indeed, members of the Prophet's broader community were not extinguished by some combination of a singular great mortality and the swords of their enemies. And yet, the hadith on the "the sword and the plague" states that all of them will perish through battle and a singular great mortality.[27] Thus, the latter meaning of "community" must signify the Companions, because God chose martyrdom in his path during battle for most of them, and the remainder perished by the plague that occurred during their time. For this reason, God combined

> death through both phenomena in them—"the sword *and* the plague"—thus the "and" keeps its primary meaning of denoting combination. It is possible that the *or* version—"the sword *or* the plague"—is valid, by indicating the variety of ways the Companions died as opposed to denoting exclusive choice.[28]

One objection to this interpretation argues that a large group of the Companions died from something other than by their enemies' swords or the plague. But the objection does not work. After all, if one can accept that it is possible to use the presumptively general sense of the term "community" to actually refer to the Companions, one must also accept that it is possible to use the term "Companions" to refer to a particular group of them.

Among the fringe interpretations of the phrase "my community" is that it refers to the community of those "called upon" to convert to Islam. Badr al-Dīn al-Zarkashī included this opinion in a volume in which he compiled a number of opinions on the plague. He asserted that:

> It is possible—and God knows best—that the intention behind the term "community" refers to the community called upon to convert to Islam, not the community who answered God's call. The evidence that is cited for this interpretation is what was already mentioned: that the cause of the plague is the appearance of grossly immoral behavior.

In my view, this definition of the term "community" is far-fetched. In fact, it is plain to see that it runs into the same problem as with the first interpretation: that most of the community called upon to convert did not die on the battlefield or by plague. Another flaw in defining "community" in this way is the fact that the appearance of grossly immoral behavior is not unique to the community of those "called upon," but it is also shared by some of the community of those who answered the call is yet another flaw in defining "community" in this way is that one of the variants of the hadith that we saw earlier with the phrase "killed in Your path" shows that the group intended here is the community that answered the call.[29] It may be correct if one were to say that the meaning of "my community" refers to a group that is broader than either those called upon to convert and those who responded affirmatively to the call, God willing, the coming discussion strengthens this view.

Al-Jaṣṣāṣ notes the following in his book *The Rulings of the Qur'an*:

> Abū Bakr al-Ṣiddīq, when he equipped the armies for battle in Damascus, prayed out, "O God, let them die by the sword or the plague."

When the plague struck Kufa, al-Mughīra ibn Shuʿba said:

> "This punishment that was foretold has now occurred. Flee from it!"

Al-Mughīra said that he mentioned that to Abū Mūsā, who replied:

> "The righteous servant Abū Bakr al-Ṣiddīq said to me: 'O God, may both the sword and the plague please you!'"[30]

This supports what I discussed earlier—that the group the Prophet intended by the phrase "my community" is the Companions.

By combining these two reports, we can see that the saying attributed to Abū Bakr in this hadith of Abū Mūsā—"O God, may both the sword and the plague please you!"—was a prayer said by him for armies that he equipped for battle. It is almost as if, when he saw them standing there at attention, he feared they would fall into civil strife. So he preferred that they go to their deaths as they went off to war before they fell into civil strife over worldly gain. Al-Jaṣṣās remarked on this hadith in his book *The Rulings of the Qur'an* that it is as if Abū Bakr al-Ṣiddīq heard the hadith from the Prophet himself, so he took consolation in it.

Shaykh Ibn Taymiyya thought al-Manbijī's citation of the

interpretation, found in his volume on the plague, of the phrase "make the end of my community . . ." as referring only to the Companions, was far-fetched. He noted that if that point were conceded, it would apply to every hadith with the phrase "the community" in it.

The truth is that initially the Prophet's call was directed at the Companions. But there is no denying the aforementioned merit to people other than the Companions. But God knows best.

Ibn Taymiyya held that construing the hadith as referring to the entire community does not contradict the hadith of Abū Mālik al-Ashʿarī, in which he states that the Prophet of God said: "God will protect you from three things: your Prophet cursing you so that you perish altogether; those who follow falsehood vanquishing those who follow the truth; and all of you coming to agreement on an error."[31]

Ibn Taymiyya did not elaborate further on why there is no contradiction. Perhaps he meant what we discussed earlier concerning the interpretation of "my community" in a narrow way, even if it is expressed in general terms.[32] Alternatively, one could say the Prophet's prayer to God that his community meet their ends "by the sword and the plague" is not a curse upon them wishing for their destruction. Rather, if they must perish, his wish in that case is that they would all achieve the status of martyr through one of those two ways. In this interpretation, when death occurs by one of those ways, it does not occur universally to all the believers in every country. If that were to occur, all the believers would vanish from the earth. Instead, it occurs only gradually, to a lesser or greater extent, whether it is through the spears of battle or the spears of the pestilence. But God knows best.

In addition, what supports construing the saying "Oh Lord! Make the end of my community . . ." as referring to the Companions is the hadith from ʿAwf ibn Mālik al-Ashjaʿī, who said:

> I went to the Prophet's place and greeted him.
> "Come in!" he said.
> "All the way in or just part of the way in?"
> "No, all of the way in . . ." he told me. "Listen, ʿAwf. . . .

> Six signs will occur as the final hour approaches. . . . The first is my death."
>
> I almost burst into tears. He stopped me.
>
> "I have only told you the first!" He continued: "The second is the conquest of the holy temple in Jerusalem. . . . The third is a mortal disease that will take my community, like the deadly Quʿāṣ disease among sheep or goats. . . . The fourth is the civil war in my community." He stressed this last one.
>
> "The fifth is that wealth will overflow among you, to the point that a person given a hundred dinārs will be discontent with it. . . . The sixth is a truce between you and the sons of Rome; then they will march eighty banners against you."
>
> "What are the banners?" I asked.
>
> "The flags . . . under each flag there are twelve thousand marching. When that day comes, the Muslims will be encamped in a land called al-Ghūṭa, in a city called Damascus."[33]

I discussed this further in my commentary on al-Bukhārī's collection, where I remarked that ʿAwf ibn Mālik spoke the Prophet's words during the Plague of ʿAmwās:

> "Count six signs as the final hour approaches. . . . Three have already occurred." He meant the Prophet's death, the conquest of the holy temple in Jerusalem, and the plague. ʿAwf added: "Three remain." Muʿādh said: "They will occur in due time. . . ."

The excesses of wealth occurred in the time of ʿUthmān, and the great civil wars started with his murder. The sixth sign has, to this day, not yet occurred.[34] This is confirmed by the hadith of the Messenger of God that said: "Fighting is sufficient for my Companions."[35]

It is as if the Prophet prayed to God to bring them that end, to obtain for them an elevation in heavenly status and to atone for their mistakes. What can be gained from this is that there is merit in dying from the plague. This is on account of the knowledge that the Prophet did not choose anything for his Companions except that which is desirable and through which the rewards of the hereafter may be gained. But God knows best.

2.5

"Your Enemies" or "Your Brothers" Among the Jinn?

All of what has been related to us by the narrations of the hadiths on the "pricks of the jinn," whether from Abū Mūsā or ʿĀʾishā or Ibn ʿUmar, are expressed with either the phrase "the pricks of your enemies" among the jinn or the phrase "the piercings of your enemies" among the jinn. Another variation in the phrasing has become well-known as well: "the pricks of your brothers" among the jinn.

I saw the following in Shaykh Badr al-Dīn al-Zarkashī's booklet:

> ʿAbdullāh ibn al-Ḥārith cited Abū Mūsā al-Ashʿarī, that he heard God's Messenger say: "The end of my community will be by the sword and the plague." They responded, "We understand 'the sword,' but what is 'the plague'?" He replied, "The piercings of your enemies among the jinn, and there is martyrdom for both." This is the phrasing in al-Ṭabarānī's collection, but in Aḥmad's phrasing, it is the piercings of "your brothers" among the jinn.[36]

Zarkashī has made a mistake in linking either the isnad or the content of this hadith to Aḥmad. Concerning the isnad, Aḥmad did not record the hadith from ʿAbdullāh ibn al-Ḥārith; rather, he transmitted it by way of three other isnads.[37] As for the content of the hadith, none of these three isnads contain the phrasing "your brothers" among the jinn at all. Rather, they contain the phrasing "your enemies" among the jinn.[38] I have no idea where al-Zarkashī found this phrase "your brothers" in Aḥmad's *Chained Hadith*, since what is found there is the phrase "your enemies."[39]

True, the jinn are described as brothers of humankind in other hadiths that have been authenticated. For instance, Muslim recorded one such hadith from ʿĀmir al-Shaʿbī's narration, in which he said: "I asked ʿAlqama, 'Was Ibn Masʿūd present with the Messenger of God the night he met and recited the Qur'an to the jinn?'" Near the end of that hadith, the jinn asked the Messenger about their provisions, and he replied:

> "Your provisions are that every bone that you find—upon which God's name was recited—will be covered in meat, and animal dung will become fodder for your riding animals." To his Companions, the Messenger said, "So do not use these items to clean yourselves after relieving yourselves, for they are the food of your brothers among the jinn."[40]

Al-Suhaylī records the following reconciliation of the two narrations by one scholar: "The first are the piercings of the believers among the jinn; the second are the piercings of the unbelievers among the jinn." This would be fine if there was a separate isnad that recorded this different version of the hadith containing the phrase "brothers of the jinn"; it does not work if both versions claim to have an identical isnad. But God knows best.

ANOTHER WAY OF UNDERSTANDING THE PLAGUE AS PRICKS OF THE JINN

Al-Zamakhsharī mentioned the following about Muʿādh in his book *The Boundless*:

> When they came from Yemen and the plague struck, ʿAmr ibn al-ʿĀṣ said: "I saw it as a punishment (rijz) from God and as a quick and wide-spreading death." It was also related

> that he said, "It was simply the result of the Devil's pricking." So Mu'ādh said, "It is neither a punishment nor a quick and wide-spreading death. It is a mercy from your Lord and the request of your Prophet. . . ."

Al-Zamakhsharī notes that the terms "al-rijz" and "al-rijs" both mean punishment. He then cited one scholar of the Arabic language who defined it as a harsh command that descends upon a people based on the following attestation: "The heavens rumbled and were menacing with thunder. The thunder is a disturbance that causes a clamor, because a punishment that descends upon a people stirs up a great commotion and panic."[41]

The broader context of the Mu'ādh hadith will be discussed in chapter four, but I did not happen upon the variant that has the phrase "the Devil's pricking" again until I found it in the *Source of the Reports* by Abū Muḥammad ibn Qutayba. In that book, he said, "The Arabs call the plague the spears of the jinn." In my opinion, this view may have originated from the early Muslim Bedouin who encountered the term for plague as coming from the Prophet. For if it had been known at the time by the pre-Islamic Arabs, why did the Companions need to ask the Prophet about its meaning, as we saw in Abū Mūsā's hadith? One possible explanation is that they asked him about the meaning of that word because it was not in their vocabulary—but God knows best.

RECONCILING THE PHRASES "PRICKS OF YOUR ENEMIES" AND "PRICKS OF YOUR BROTHERS," ASSUMING THAT BOTH ARE AUTHENTIC

I have seen five ways of harmonizing these two phrases. The first approach is mentioned by al-Shiblī, whose opinions were noted. He argued, "There is no contradiction between the two phrasings, because being brothers in religion does not exclude them from also being enemies, since the jinn are enemies to humankind by nature. Even if those jinn are believers, enmity still exists." It is possible to cite, as a proof-text, the words of God in the Qur'an, which addresses humankind's origin—Adam and Eve—and the jinn's origin—Iblīs:* "We said, 'Go down from here as enemies to one another.'"[42] Another would be the words of God to humankind about Iblīs: "So do you then take him and his offspring as protectors instead of Me, despite their enmity toward you?"[43]

The heart of this explanation is that the jinn are described at their core as enemies of humankind, regardless of whether they are believers or unbelievers. It is as if al-Shiblī held the expression "your enemies" as problematic and composed a response for it while affirming the phrase "your brother," without regarding it as a problem, and hence not attempting to explain it. But this is contrary to how others understand the issue.

Al-Zarkashī noted:

> If both narrations are correct, it may be possible—and God knows best how to harmonize them—that the narration that contains "your enemies" is referring to the unbelievers among the jinn and their pricking upon the Muslims of humankind. Meanwhile, the narration that contains "your brothers" is the pricks of the Muslims among them upon the unbelievers of humankind.[44]

This way of harmonizing these two phrasings would work, except that it requires the meaning of each narration to refer only to a distinct group. This would work more easily if the isnads recorded by the collector were different, since they could be interpreted as two separate hadiths. However, they share the same isnad, and that link therefore suggests that the disagreement lies in the phrasing of some of its narrators of the same hadith. If this were not so, the collector would have cited it

*Iblīs often identified with Satan, whom, according to the Qur'an, God cast into the fire when he refused to bow to Adam; the Qur'an suggests Iblīs is related to the jinn or created from the same substance (Qur'an 18:50).

with both phrases together at least once, in order to validate them both.

I heard of a third approach involving Ibn Kathīr, who was asked about this issue and answered it in the following way: The narration with the phrasing that claims that the piercings of the plague are from "your enemies among the jinn" is interpreted as referring to direct contact as the proximate cause of the piercings, and the narrations that the piercings of the plague are from "your brothers among the jinn" refers to the indirect cause. This explanation proceeds on the grounds that the ones addressed "as brothers among the jinn" are believers exclusively, and that it is the unbelievers among the jinn that exclusively pierce humankind. Sometimes the unbelieving jinn merely has enmity for a person, and that unbelieving jinn directly pierces that believer. However, sometimes the unbelieving jinn pierces a person on account of a struggle between the believing jinn and the unbelieving jinn. Take, for instance, an unbelieving jinn who is unable to oppose the believing jinn. The unbelieving jinn then takes vengeance by piercing a person who is a believer. So it can be said that the believing jinn is the indirect cause of the striking of the plague upon the believing person.

Ibn Kathīr offered the words of God—"Do not curse those unbelievers who call upon idols instead of God, lest they revile God out of spite and ignorance"[45]—as further proof of the validity of this theory of indirect causality in order to harmonize these two versions of the hadith. He also cited the following hadith as a proof-text. It warned against cursing another man's father:

> "How is it possible to curse one's own father?" they asked.
>
> The Prophet replied, "If one curses the father of another man, that man curses his father in return."

In my view, this third approach to harmonizing the two phrasings would also work, were it not for what we explained in response to the second approach—that the two versions share the same isnad.

A fourth approach occurred to me, and I have not seen it cited anywhere. It views the variation in phrasing as the result of the hadith's narrators in a way that comports with the hadith's singular recorded isnad, as we discussed earlier. It is based on the notion that the two phrasings are interchangeable in terms of their meaning. If we assume this, the phrasing "the piercings of the plague are the pricks of your enemies among the jinn" encompasses the totality of everyone. This is because the piercing does not strike except between enemies, so the phrasing addresses all humankind and all jinn: the unbelievers among the jinn who strike the believers of humankind and the believers of the jinn who strike the unbelievers of humankind. A prooftext that supports this interpretation is the hadith of Abū ʿAsīb, which we have seen, that states that the plague was martyrdom for the believers and a punishment for the unbelievers.

Meanwhile, the phrasing "the piercings of the plague are the pricks of your brothers among the jinn" also refers to the totality of everyone. However, the meaning of "brothers" here refers to a "brotherhood" of corresponding pairs, as in "night and day are brothers" and "the sun and the moon are brothers." Or it could refer to the brotherhood of moral responsibility, for both the humans and the jinn are two burdened species according to the Qur'an, because both of them are subject to moral responsibility.

Ibn ʿAbd al-Barr, in his book *The Easy Path Forward*, wrote: "The majority of religious scholars consider the jinn to be subject to moral responsibility and addressed by the Divine revelation." Ibn Ḥazm said in his book *The Sects*:

> Definitive scripture affirms the notion that the jinn are a community who can reason; are capable of rational discrimination; are subject to moral responsibility; have been promised reward and threatened with punishment by God; have progeny and die. All of the Muslims have come to consensus on this point. Indeed, even the Christians, the Magians, and the Jews have as well. Only the Samaritans are the exception.

Imām Fakhr al-Dīn al-Rāzī added this in his commentary on the Qur'an: "Everyone, that is, those that affirm the existence of the jinn, agree that the jinn are responsible moral agents."

It certainly is the case that the phrase "your brothers among the jinn" encompasses all jinn when viewed from this perspective. It would be correct to describe those who pierce humankind in that way, as is the case with the phrase "the enemies among the jinn." This is the proper reply to the hadith about the time that the Prophet was asked about the provisions God supplied for the jinn, which contains the phrase "your brothers among the jinn" in all of its isnads, and not the phrase "your enemies among the jinn." What is intended by that word "brothers" in the hadith are all kinds of the jinn—believers and unbelievers—for they share in bones and dung being their provisions. But God knows best.

The essence of this view is cited in a volume that Abū 'Abdullāh al-Manbijī al-Ṣāliḥī al-Ḥanbalī put together on the plague:

> One of the later scholars held, "The intent is not brotherhood in religion. Rather, the intent is the brotherhood of corresponding pairs. For the humans and the jinn are corresponding pairs because they are both regarded as species burdened with responsibility." The above is his wording. And God knows best.

One of the early Qur'anic exegetes said, commenting on the verse "O sister of Aaron":

> The verse means the brotherhood of similarity and not lineage: There was in that time a man called Aaron who was either "righteous" or "evil," based on the difference in the narrations, and they regarded her as similar to him.[46]

It is possible that this is what is meant in our case—that the jinn and the humans are similar to each other in their capacity to bear moral responsibility, as we saw.

The fifth approach to reconciling the two phrases is what one esteemed scholar remarked to me: that the phrase in the narration "the pricking of your enemies" is construed with respect to the agent, and the phrase "your brothers" with respect to the one being acted upon. This means that the first phrasing—"your enemies"—refers to that which jinn do to people, and the second—"your brothers"—to that which befalls the believers among the jinn. It is plain to see that this way of reconciling the two phrases is strained and unlikely to be correct.

It is possible to establish a sixth approach, based on the meaning of the last hadith that I mention at the end of chapter three, so one may review it there.

THE MEANING OF "THERE IS MARTYRDOM FOR EACH" PERSON WHO DIES OF PLAGUE

A problem occurred to me regarding a sinner who dies of the plague. What is the ruling on his status in the afterlife? To which of the two groups does he belong? By sinner, I mean one who commits grave sins. When such a person is struck by the plague while he is resolute in his disobedience to God, does he still die a martyr?

There are some who say that such a sinner would not receive the honor of martyrdom, on account of his wicked acts, for God, may He be exalted, spoke these words in the Qur'an: "Do those who commit wicked acts reckon that We shall deal with them in the same way as We deal with those who are faithful and do good works? That they will be alike in their living and their dying? How badly they judge!"[47]

But one may also say that he has achieved the martyr's status. Why? Because the existing reports on the plague that confer martyrdom make no such exclusion. This type of martyrdom is awarded to a Muslim for something that goes beyond their particular observance of Islam. This idea is also found in many hadiths; among them is Anas's hadith in the *Authentic Hadith* of both al-Bukhārī and Muslim: "The plague offers martyrdom for every Muslim." It is clear and explicit in the generality of its application.

Of course, it is not necessarily the case that he who has done wicked things and still obtains martyrdom is equal in station to the believer who does good deeds, as the status of martyrs occurs in degrees. The sinner who dies of plague and thus becomes a martyr is at the level of a believing sinner who kills non-believers fighting in God's cause. That is, they are like a sinner who fights in order to elevate God's word, being steadfast in battle and not retreating—such a person is definitely a martyr even if he has sins for which he has not yet repented. In the third chapter, we will see ʿUtba ibn ʿAbd's hadith clearly states that God effaces the missteps of anyone who commits sins and errs but sacrifices himself in jihad with his person and his wealth, for the sword is the effacer of sins.

Indeed, all of the martyr's sins are forgiven except a financial debt owed to another human being, as the authentic hadith establishes; and all obligations owed to others are included in the meaning of "debt."

Let us also respond to what God's Messenger was said to have said: "The martyr at sea is like two martyrs on land. . . . While the martyr on land is forgiven for all of his sins except debt, the martyr at sea is forgiven for his sins and his debt."[48] If this were proven to be authentic, then it would be specific to a pious warrior who leaves home and dies by drowning, because he combines two grounds for martyrdom: fighting in the path of God and drowning.

One can also say that the debt exemption in the hadith affirms the principle that obligations owed to others cannot be canceled solely by obtaining martyrdom. The rest of the hadith shows that God, the Exalted, has gifted the martyr with so much heavenly reward on account of his martyrdom that the martyr may transfer his good deeds to others in order to fulfill any obligations he owes them due to an injustice on his part. Martyrdom's heavenly reward alone more than suffices for him.

The main point of this is that the existence of obligations due to others does not prevent one from obtaining martyrdom. This is because the Lawgiver has made heavenly reward a consequence of a certain quality, so that when it is attained for the believer at death, he has attained the heavenly reward as a grace from God and an act of benevolence and fulfillment of God's promise—for God does not go back on what He promises. The only meaning martyrdom has is that the Exalted rewards one who obtains it with a certain heavenly reward and honors him with an additional distinction.

The hadith clarifies that God expiates sins connected with duties owed to Him, and He overlooks those that neglect them by omitting punishment for them. If it is assumed that the martyr has done good deeds and that martyrdom has expiated evil acts not connected to duties owed to human beings, then his good deeds will benefit him when weighed against what he owes others, and they will be satisfied by these good deeds by way of a gift from God and through His mercy.

Attaining martyrdom does not require canceling duties owed to other human beings. The absence of duties owed to others in the case of one who is free from such debts stems from the necessity of his life on earth and not from the logic of recompense for martyrdom. An example of this is when one of the king's intimate friends wrongs another one of his friends. The king punishes his first friend out of respect for the other's rights, yet this does not negate his esteem for the one he punishes. On the contrary, it is often the case that he goes to great lengths to honor this particular friend of his, because he fulfills, on his friend's behalf, the claims that those outside his circle may have over him, choosing both justice and love in the service of equity. How can this not be the case with God, who "does not wrong by as much as an atom's weight; and if there be a good deed, He will multiply it."[49]

Thus, through this account one knows that the wisdom of the exception found in the phrase "except debt" in the hadith indicates the existence of a distinction between the one who has no worldly obligations, not requiring the conferral of graces in the heavenly reward for martyrdom, and the one who has worldly obligations and is thereby hindered from enjoying his heavenly reward until his obligations to the relevant people are fulfilled.

In support of this, God's Messenger said:

> "When the believers attain safety from hell by crossing the path over it, they will be detained on a bridge between heaven and hell. The injustices that occurred between them in this world will be litigated, until they have been cleansed and purified. Then they will be permitted to enter the heavenly garden. . . ."[50]

So there can be no doubt that the ranking of those who are detained on the bridge between heaven and hell is lower than those who are permitted to enter the heavenly garden without impediment.

ANSWERS TO THE PROBLEMS POSED BY "THE PLAGUE IS FROM THE PRICKS OF THE JINN"

Al-Subkī said:

> If the hadith of Abū Mūsā on the plague is correct, it requires that the plague not occur during the month of Ramadan, because the demons are bound and shackled during that month, as is established in al-Bukhārī's *Authentic Hadith*. However, why is it that not only has the plague occurred during this month, but we have observed it occur more frequently during this month than others?
>
> There is nothing in the hadith that suggests that the demons' activities are completely stopped. Rather, one can take from the hadith that just the better part of their activity is prevented. . . . It is also possible for some to say that the demons pierce people prior to the beginning of the month of Ramadan, but the effects do not appear until after its start. But this is unlikely to be the case.
>
> It occurred to me that one could say that the demons are only shackled from enticing humans in committing acts

> that entail sin. As for those matters that do not result in sin but instead offer opportunities for a person to be rewarded, such as the plague, demons are not obstructed from such activity. In the same way, demons are not prevented from those activities that result in neither sin nor reward, such as inspiring wet dreams.

The learned scholars of old discussed this problem. They problematized the notion of shackling demons during Ramadan in another way: How does one explain the existence of disobedience, even grave sins, and other things that human beings commit during the holy month? ʿAbdullāh ibn Aḥmad said:

> I asked my father about this hadith that says the demons are shackled during Ramadan: "Yet man still experiences the demon's whispering and is brought down!" His father replied: "So says the hadith."

I have written extensively on this issue in my book *Fath al-Bārī* (The Divine Aid to Victory). This is what I wrote, in short: Al-Ḥalīmī notes:

> It is possible that those shackled are the demons that eavesdrop in the heavens trying to pilfer news of the unseen. Their being shackled occurs during the nights of Ramadan, and not its days, because they were absolutely prevented from eavesdropping on the descent of the Qur'an during Ramadan and other months, in order to effectively safeguard revelation. It is also possible that it means that during Ramadan the demons are not dedicated to corrupting Muslims in the way they are in other months of the year, because Muslims are occupying themselves with fasting, which represses the desire to act on temptations, as well as reciting the Qur'an, remembering God, and prayer.

Ibn Khuzayma said: "The meaning of the hadith refers to some of the demons but not all." For this reason, Ibn Khuzayma arranged a section on it in his *Authentic Hadith*. I cite what he recorded, with his phrasing: Abū Hurayra said the Prophet said: "When the first night of Ramadan occurs, the demons will be shackled without chains." In al-Tirmidhī's narration, "The demons and the evil jinn are shackled." The word "and" indicates a conjunction. Al-Nasāʾī has another version from Abū Hurayra with the following phrasing: "The rebellious demons are shackled during Ramadan."[51] The unqualified term in the narrations in Ibn Khuzayma's *Authentic Hadith* should be read as qualified by the term "rebellious," thus excluding those demons who are not rebellious. It is possible to reconcile them by saying that the pricking that happens during Ramadan is from the non-evil spirits.

Qāḍī ʿIyāḍ said:

> It is possible to interpret the shackling of the demons in two ways. First, it is interpreted according to its apparent and literal sense: the demons are prevented from physically harming the believers. It is also possible to interpret it as an indication of the increase in heavenly reward, and that the demons' deceptions are diminished so that they become like those who are enfettered. This is thus a metaphor for their inability to deceive people and make the people's vulgar desires alluring to them.

Al-Qurṭubī preferred interpreting it in its apparent and literal sense in his *Book of Discerning*. He said:

> If someone were to object: If the demons are shackled, how can much evil and sin be seen to occur in the month of Ramadan? Why do evil deeds occur at that time? The answer is the following: First, the demons are only shackled from the one who fasts while properly observing its conditions and paying attention to its proper etiquette. Second, those spirits who are shackled are only some of them—the evil ones—not all of them. Third, it refers to the decrease of evil deeds during Ramadan, since the existence of evil during that month is observably less than in other months.

The best of these three possibilities is the second, on the basis of what we discussed earlier concerning the variant hadiths, and because it best overcomes the objection—but God knows best.

2.6

Being Possessed by a Jinn

The following hadiths are cited as proof that the jinn enjoy power over humankind without pricking them during Ramadan and other months. This evidence does not repudiate the fact that the jinn also subjugate humankind through the pricks of their spears, or the fact that God uses some jinn to repel other jinn.

The Prophet said: "Satan flows through Adam's descendants, like blood" flows through their veins; this is established in the *Authentic Hadith* of al-Bukhārī and Muslim, citing Ṣafiyya bint Ḥuyayy, the mother of the believers, as she told the story of the Prophet's seclusion during Ramadan. Although in this context it refers in particular to the Devil, who whispers temptations in people's ears, the phrasing allows the possibility of signifying something generalizable to the jinn. Moreover, the empirical evidence of jinn possessing human beings is very large.

Al-Bazzār records the following hadith from Samura, which he attributes directly to the Prophet:

> "Satan has kohl and an electuary.* When he applies kohl to a man, he keeps him busy from prayer. When he feeds a

*Kohl is a kind of black eye makeup; an electuary is a sweet medicinal syrup.

man his electuary, the man's tongue gains eloquence in speaking evil."[52]

Ibn Abī al-Dunyā reported the following in the book *The Devil's Traps*, with an authentic isnad, related from the Companion Anas, that stated:

> No sooner had the daughter of ʿAwf ibn ʿAfrāʾ lay down on her bed, when she felt a man from among the Zanj leap upon her chest and place his hand on her throat.* She said, "Suddenly a leaf of paper fell from the sky toward the earth until it landed on my chest—so he took it and read it. Here is what it said: 'From Lukayn's Lord to Lukayn: Avoid the daughter of the righteous man, for you have no right to take action against her.' So he stood up and released his hand from my throat and struck my knee with it, and it began to swell until it was shaped like a sheep's head. So I went to ʿĀʾisha, and I told her what happened. She replied, 'Niece of mine! When you start menstruating, dress modestly; God willing, he will not be able to harm you anymore.'" God protected her on account of her father, for he died as a martyr in the battle of Badr.†[53]

*Zanj is a region in East Africa, typically associated with the Swahili coast or near modern-day Zanzibar; the term is sometimes infelicitously employed in Arabic literature to refer to anyone with a black complexion.

†The Battle of Badr, a watershed victory for Muhammad against his opponents, was said to have taken place during Ramadan of 624 CE.

2.7

The Wisdom Behind the Jinn's Subjugation of Humanity Through the Plague

Ibn al-Qayyim says:

> There is profound wisdom in the plague being the result of the pricks of our enemies from among the jinn. This is because our enemies among them are demons. As for those among the jinn who are obedient to God, they are our brothers. God commanded us to oppose our enemies among the jinn and humankind, demanding that we combat them for His satisfaction. But most people refused to do anything except appease them. Because people listened to and obeyed those demons when they misguided them, ordered them to sin, live immorally, and sow chaos in the land, God gave the jinn power to punish them. Divine wisdom requires that the jinn are empowered to wound them, just as he gave their human enemies power over them when they sowed chaos in the land and in defiance cast God's book aside. The latter is the war undertaken by people, and the plague is the war undertaken by the jinn. Each one was empowered by God—the Most High and the Supremely Wise—as a punishment for those who deserve it, and as a martyrdom and a mercy for those who are worthy of it. This is God's practice in the matter of punishments that befall the general populace. Divine punishments purify the believers and exact retribution from the wicked.

We shall see abundant examples supporting this argument in chapter three, God willing. But I will now mention a different piece of wisdom related to this issue that Ibn al-Qayyim did not point out.

Al-Kalābādhī, in *The Meaning of the Reports*, notes:

> God, the most High and Exalted, chose the individual believer for Himself, directing His attention to him alone in showing him love, making all of his circumstances the best for him, willing him the best in everything that touches him, whether that be hardship, fortune, pain, or pleasure. God wills the good for him when He sends him someone who would support him—the angel who seeks forgiveness for him and the Prophet who intercedes for him and the fellow believer who assists him. God also wills the good for him when He makes someone who harbors enmity for him—Satan who humiliates him, an enemy who fights with him, and a jinn who wounds him. And He, the most High and Exalted, is a Protector and Champion for the believer and a humiliating Vanquisher of his enemies. The believer is he who, when struck with fortune, gives thanks, which is the best for him; and if he is struck with hardship, then he is patient, which is the best for him.

Then al-Kalābādhī discussed his response to the problem of the jinn having power over the believer, even as the believer is protected by God in all affairs. He wrote:

> It is like when God permits the believer's clear enemy to wound him with a spear and a sword, despite the fact that most of the time God prevents his enemy from doing so, occasionally through inspiring fear, and other times through force and conquest. When his enemy kills him, God wills good through it and confers the status of a martyr upon him. It is likewise the case when the enemy seizes the territory and wealth of a Muslim, despite God's words: "You will be the most exalted, if you are believers," and His words "God will never make a path to victory for the unbelievers over the believers."[54] And in just this way, God permitted the enemies from among the jinn to wound a believer, despite the fact that most of the time God prevents the jinn

> from doing so through the agency of the angels. However, when He allows it, He wills the best by it, and confers the status of the martyr upon them. So it is also possible in the prick of a jinn's spear, despite the Most High's declaration: "Satan's plot is weak."[55]

The thrust of a person's spear penetrates the body, while the thrust of a jinn's spear does not penetrate. The Prophet called a penetrating spear ṭaʿn, and he called one that does not penetrate ṭāʿūn, or "piercings" of the plague, and declared that either one can result in attaining martyrdom.

AN EYEWITNESS ACCOUNT OF A JINN STRIKING A HORSE WITH PLAGUE

It is related in numerous corroborating accounts and stories that the plague is the result of the pricking of the jinn. Most recently, al-Sharīf Shihāb al-Dīn ibn ʿAdnān, who was the chief secretary* in Cairo at the time, reports the following story. I think I may have heard this from him directly and read about it from the hand of someone I trust. He said:

> One time, the plague took hold, so I went to visit the sick.
>
> "Pierce him with plague," I heard someone whisper to another.
>
> "No . . ." the other said. "No!"
>
> "In that case, leave him be. He might be of use to the people."
>
> "True."
>
> "Fine. Then in his horse's eye!"
>
> After hearing that, I whipped around to see who was whispering. I didn't see anyone. So I visited the sick. On my

*The office of the chief secretary, or Kātib al-Sirr, was the head of the chancery and was traditionally considered the most influential and senior adviser to the sultan in Cairo during the Mamluk Sultanate.

way back, I suddenly saw a horse who had escaped from its riders. They had tracked it down in order to bring it back. Its eye had vanished without a perceptible trace of a beating. Since then, I have sworn that the saying "The plague is from the pricks of the jinn" is true. I used to have my doubts!

2.8

The Formulae to Recite to Protect One from the Jinn's Ploys

CHAPTERS AND VERSES FROM THE QUR'AN TO RECITE THAT WILL PROTECT ONE FROM THE JINN

The opening chapter of the Qur'an—called the Fātiḥa—is recommended for seeking protection and healing.[56] Similarly, God's Messenger said the following about the opening chapter of the Qur'an:

> "It is a cure for every illness."[57]

God's Messenger said:

> "If you lie down on the bed on your side and read the opening chapter of the Qur'an and the chapter near the end of the Qur'an that begins 'Say: God is One,' then you will be protected from everything except death."[58]

God's Messenger said:

> "The Devil flees from the house in which the Qur'an's Chapter of the Cow is recited."[59]

God's Messenger said:

> "The Chapter of the Cow has a verse that is the chief verse of the Qur'an—the Throne verse.* If a house is possessed by the Devil, no sooner is that verse read than the Devil flees from it."[60]

The Prophet also said:

> "God wrote a book two thousand years before he created the heavens and the earth, and from it He sent down two verses that conclude the Chapter of the Cow. The Devil approaches dwellings in which they are not recited for three nights."[61]

There is also the report from Ibn Mas'ūd, who said:

> "Whoever recites the following ten verses from the Chapter of the Cow, the Devil will not enter their house that night until daybreak: the four verses at the beginning of the chapter, the Throne verse and two verses that follow it, and the three closing verses of the chapter."[62]

According to the hadith from Abū Hurayra, which begins with the phrase "God's Messenger entrusted to me the duty to collect the alms-tax of Ramadan," there is a phrase in which a jinn spoke these words to Abū Hurayra:

> When you go to bed, recite the Throne verse—"God: there is no god but Him, the Living, the Eternal . . . " until the

---

*The Throne verse is Qur'an 2:255: "God: there is no god but Him, the Living, the Eternal. Neither slumber nor sleep overtakes Him. To Him belongs that which is in the heavens and the earth. Who can intercede with Him except by His permission? He knows all that is before them and all that is behind them. They can grasp only that part of His knowledge which He wills. His throne extends over the heavens and the earth; and protecting them both does not tire Him. He is the Sublime, the Almighty One!"

> end of the verse—for then a Protector from God will continuously watch over you, and Satan will not approach you until daybreak.
>
> The Prophet said: "He speaks the truth to you, though he is normally a liar."[63]

As stated in the hadith citing Abū Ayyūb al-Anṣārī:

> Abū Ayyūb used to have a little shack that stored dates. A ghoul used to come and snatch dates from it.
>
> The ghoul said to Abū Ayyūb: "The Throne verse . . . if you recite it in your home, neither the Devil nor anything else will approach you."
>
> Abū Ayyūb told the Prophet about this.
>
> "She speaks the truth to you," the Prophet said. "Even though she is a liar."[64]

There is a hadith from Ubayy ibn Kaʿb, recorded by al-Nasāʾī and Abū Yaʿlā, which states that he used to have a barn house that stored dates. The hadith continued:

> Suddenly, Ubayy's riding animal took the form of a full-grown manservant.
>
> "What are you?" Ubayy exclaimed.
>
> "I am a jinn . . ."
>
> "What will protect us from your kind?"
>
> "The Throne verse . . ."
>
> Later, the Prophet said: "That evil thing spoke the truth."

In a hadith cited by Burayda, he said, "I heard that Muʿādh ibn Jabal took hold of Satan during the time of God's Messenger. So I asked him, and he confirmed it." Then Burayda continued with this hadith:

> The jinn took the form of an elephant, and entered through a crack in the door, and approached the dates. . . .
>
> "We used to be in this city of yours!" said the jinn. "That

is, until your companion Muhammad was sent. When two particular verses were revealed to him, we grew afraid of the verses because we fell under their power. Satan will never enter the house for three nights in which these two verses are recited: the Throne verse and the concluding verses of the Cow Chapter, starting with 'The Messenger believes . . .' until the end."

I then released the jinn and made my way to God's Messenger the next morning.

"He has spoken the truth," the Messenger of God said. "Even though he is a liar."[65]

The Prophet also said:

"There is a verse in the Qur'an's Chapter of the Cow, such that if it is recited the demons disperse from a home. If it is not recited, Satan enters it."[66]

There is also a hadith from Kaʿb al-Aḥbār in which he says:

Muhammad was given four verses that Moses was not given, and Moses was given a verse that Muhammad was not given. The verses are: the Throne verse till the end of the Cow Chapter. The verse given to Moses was: "O God, do not allow Satan to enter our hearts, and purify us of him. To you belong sovereignty, strength, power, kingship, praise, the heavens, the earth, and destiny, eternally and always."[67]

Muḥammad ibn al-Mundhir al-Harawī recorded the following in his book *The Wonders*, attributed to Ḥamza al-Zayyāt:

When I was in Helwan—in Egypt—I heard one demon talking to another demon.

"That thing which people recite is the Qur'an—come, let's amuse ourselves and have some fun with it!"

"That is a recipe for disaster," said the other demon.

When they approached me, I recited: "God bears witness that there is no God but Him, as do the angels and those who possess knowledge."[68]

"The power of God compels me," said one to the other. "I will stay to protect him until the rising of the sun."

Ubayy ibn Kaʿb said:

I was with the Prophet when a Bedouin arrived.

"Prophet of God! I have a brother who is sick."

"What kind of ailment?"

"He is mentally ill."

"Bring him to me."

The Bedouin brought his brother to the Prophet, who recited the following sections from the Qur'an: the opening chapter; four verses from the beginning of the Chapter of the Cow, as well as the verse "Your God is One," from that same chapter; the Throne verse; three verses from the end of the Chapter of the Family of ʿImrān, as well as the verse "God bears witness that there is no god but He . . ." from that same chapter; the verse from the Chapter of the Heights, "Indeed, your Lord is God"; the verse near the end of the Chapter of the Believers, "Exalted is God"; ten verses near the beginning of the Chapter of the Arrangers; three verses from the end of the Chapter of the Gathering; the verse from the Chapter of the Jinn, "He, Exalted . . ."; and the last three chapters of the Qur'an that seek refuge in God.[69]

After the Prophet recited these verses to the Bedouin's brother, he stood up as if he had never complained about anything in the first place.

The Messenger of God said:

"Whoever recites the Throne Verse and the opening verses of the Chapter of Ḥā Mīm when he rises, he is protected until evening. If he recites it in the evening, he is protected until morning."[70]

ʿUqba ibn ʿĀmir said:

> I was marching with the Messenger of God at al-Juḥfā and al-Abwāʾ when we experienced high winds and dark skies. So the Messenger of God began to recite the last two chapters of the Qur'an, seeking refuge in God.
>
> "Listen, ʿUqba!" he said. "Recite these two chapters when seeking refuge, there are no two like it."[71]

The Prophet also said:

> "Seek refuge in God by reciting 'Say: God is One,' 'Say: I seek refuge the Lord of Daybreak,' 'Say: I seek refuge in the Lord of humankind.' A servant of God cannot seek refuge in Him in any better way."[72]

A hadith from al-Nasāʾī states that ʿAbdullāh ibn Khubayb said:

> It was drizzling and dark, and we were waiting for the Prophet to lead us in prayer. At last, he came out.
>
> "Recite!" he said.
>
> "What do I recite?"
>
> "At dusk and at daybreak, recite the chapter 'Say that He is One' and the two closing chapters of the Qur'an that follow it. That will be sufficient for you in all things."[73]

Abū ʿUbayd had a hadith that cited ʿAbd al-Raḥmān ibn ʿAbbās:

> The Messenger of God said: "Ibn ʿAbbās! Did I never teach you the best way to seek refuge in God?"
>
> "No, you did not, O Messenger of God."
>
> "'Say: I seek refuge in the Lord of Daybreak'; 'Say: I seek refuge in the Lord of humankind.'"[74]

Abū Saʿīd al-Khudrī said:

> The Messenger of God used to seek protection from the jinn and the evil eye by reciting the last two chapters of the

Qur'an. When those were revealed, he seized upon them and discarded others.[75]

PRAYERS THAT WILL PROTECT ONE FROM THE JINN

God's Messenger said:

"Whoever repeats one hundred times 'There is no god but God alone, who has no partner, Kingship and praise belong to Him, He is powerful over all things,' that would be equal in merit to the act of freeing ten slaves . . . protecting him from the Devil on that day until the setting of the sun."[76]

God's Messenger said:

"If, after the morning prayer, one says, 'There is no god but God,' reciting it ten times, while his legs are still folded and before he begins his normal speech, God records ten good deeds for him, erases ten bad deeds from his record, and lifts his station by ten degrees. That day he will be secure from every reprehensible thing and protected from Satan."[77]

God's Messenger said:

"God commanded John, the son of Zechariah,* to command the children of Israel . . . to invoke God's name in repeated recitation. An analogy to this would be a person fleeing his enemies in hot pursuit, until he reaches the protection of a fortress, safeguarding himself from them. That resembles the pious servant who safeguards himself from the demons by invoking God's name in repeated recitation."[78]

---

*Known to Christians as John the Baptist.

God's Messenger said:

> "During my night journey* I saw a mischievous jinn searching for me with a torch; wherever I turned, I saw him.
>
> So the Angel Gabriel said to me: 'Did I not teach you the words to say to extinguish his torch?'
>
> I replied, 'No, you did not.'
>
> Gabriel then instructed, 'Say: "I seek refuge in God's noble countenance; I seek refuge in God's perfect words, which neither a pious person and nor a sinner can exceed; I seek refuge from the evil that descends from the sky, and from the evil that rises up to it, from the evil that He scatters across the earth, and from the evil that emerges from it, and from the trials and visitations of the night and the day, except for the visitor who comes with blessings."'"[79]

ʿAlī cites the Prophet as saying:

> "One should say 'in the name of God' when going to relieve oneself to make a veil between the jinn and the nakedness of human beings."[80]

ʿAbdullāh ibn ʿAmr said that God's Messenger used to utter the following phrase when he entered a place of worship:

> "I seek refuge in the glorious God, in His noble countenance, and in His eternal power, from the accursed Devil," and the Devil replied, "He is safeguarded from me for the rest of the day."[81]

---

*In Arabic, laylat al-isrā'; this refers to "the night journey" described in the Qur'ān to "the furthest place of worship"—a place that some associate with Heaven and others with Jerusalem (the latter is more common). In some accounts in the hadith, Muhammad is awakened from his slumber by the Angel Gabriel and ascends on the back of a winged animal called Burāq. There is scholarly debate over whether the night journey was a physical journey, a vision, or a combination of both. *The Encyclopedia of Islam,* 1st ed., eds. M. Th. Houtsma, T. W. Arnold, R. Basset, and R. Hartmann (Leiden: Brill, 1913–1936; *EI1*), (B. Schreike).

Anas ibn Mālik cited God's Messenger, saying:

> "If a man goes out from his home and says, 'In the name of God, I trust in God, and there is neither might nor power in other than God,' then it will be said to him, 'You are guided, saved, and safeguarded,' and the Devil will slink away. That Devil will say to another: 'What can you do with a man who is guided, saved, and safeguarded?'"[82]

Ibn ʿAbbās said the Prophet said:

> "These words are a remedy for every disease: 'I seek refuge in God's perfect words and each of his names all together from the evil of poisonous pests and insects, from the evil of the envious eye, from the evil of the covetous one when he covets, and from the evil of the deceitful serpent and his progeny . . .'"[83]

ʿAbdullāh ibn Masʿūd cited the Prophet, saying:

> "When one of you finds himself fearing the sultan, let him say the following three times: 'O God, Lord of the seven heavens and the tremendous throne, be, for me, a guardian from the evil of this person, from the evil of man and jinn and their followers. Protect me from the abuse of even a single one of them. May Your protection be exalted and Your praise be glorified. There is no god but You."[84]

Ibn ʿAbbās cited the Prophet, saying:

> "When you approach an intimidating sultan whose assault you fear, say the following three times: 'Allahu Akbar, God is mightier than all of His creation. God is mightier than what I fear and dread. I seek refuge in God, besides whom there is no other god, the One who keeps the heavens from collapsing on earth, which is only sustained through His will. I seek Your protection from this servant of Yours, his army, his followers, and his partisans from among the jinn

and men. O God, be for me a protector from their evil. May Your praise be glorified, Your protection exalted, and Your name be blessed. There is no god but You.'"[85]

ʿAṭāʾ ibn Abī Marwan cited his father, who said that Kaʿb swore that Ṣuhayb told him the following hadith:

> Muḥammad did not ever lay eyes upon a village that he wanted to enter without saying the following when he beheld it: "O God, Lord of the seven heavens and what casts shadows, Lord of the earths and what diminishes, Lord of the demons and what misguides, Lord of the winds and what scatters. I ask You for the good of this village and its people. I seek refuge in You from the evil of its people, and whatever is in it."[86]

Khawla bint Ḥakīm said that God's Messenger said:

> "Whoever sets up camp in a place, and says, 'I seek refuge in God's perfect words from the evil He created,' nothing will harm him until he decamps."[87]

It is often relayed that al-Walīd ibn al-Walīd ibn al-Mughīra once cried:

> "Prophet of God! I am beset with melancholy."
>
> The Prophet replied: "When you lie down, utter the following phrase: 'I seek refuge in God's perfect words from His anger and His punishment and the wickedness of His servants, and from the temptations of the demons.' If they come, they will not harm you."[88]

ʿAbdullāh ibn ʿUmar said:

> When God's Messenger traveled and came upon nightfall, he would say: "Earth! My Lord and your Lord is God. I seek refuge in God from your evil, and the evil within you, and the evil he created in you and the evil that befalls you. I

seek refuge in God from lions, serpents, snakes, scorpions, town dwellers, and the evil of what gives birth and what it births."[89]

Abū al-Asmar al-ʿAbdī said:

A man went to the outer parts of Kūfa and mentioned this story. While he was out there, he heard a jinn.

"There is no way to harm ʿUrwā ibn al-Zubayr," the jinn shouted, "because he recites religious formulae at daybreak and sunset!"

The man then went to Medina and asked Ibn al-Zubayr what he says each day to protect himself.

He said: "I recite 'I believe in God alone, I reject idols and demons, I have taken hold of an unfailing support, which breaks not, and God is All-hearing, All-wise.'"[90]

WHAT REPELS THE PLAGUE AND THE PESTILENCE, IN AL-SHĀFIʿĪ'S VIEW?

One of the manuscript copies of *The Ornament* contains an opinion attributed to al-Shāfiʿī: "The best thing to treat the plague is to recite 'Glory be to God!' repeatedly."[91] And it is said that his view was that repeated recitation of religious formulae lifts the punishment implemented by God and the destruction wrought upon them, just as God, may He be exalted, revealed in the Qur'an: "Had he not been one of those who glorified God, Jonah would have remained inside the whale until the Day of Resurrection."[92] ʿUmar once ordered that a man be flogged, but pardoned him when the man cried "Glory be to God!" after the first lash struck his skin; it was transmitted that Kaʿb al-Aḥbār, who witnessed this incident, said afterward, "Glorifying God repels punishment!"

For myself, I would note that what Ibn Abī Ḥātim and others transmitted about al-Shāfiʿī is well-known: "I have found nothing more beneficial than violets in treating the pestilence, daubing its oil and drinking it."

A WORD OF CAUTION

The benefit is achieved by reciting these verses and repeating these formulae only for the man whose heart is purified from the stain of sin and who is sincere in repentance, and full of regret for those good deeds he neglected and those sins that escaped his notice. If his heart is not pure, then the cause of the disease overpowers that which promotes healing, perhaps canceling the effectiveness of the remedy. It would have been enough, in showing the benefit of reciting these formulae, had there been no example for this phenomenon in the empirical world, but man's heedlessness of the aforementioned things is such that the disease attacks him without him perceiving it. This leads to him to seek release from its grip but instead he finds no escape from it.

So we ask God, may He be exalted, to fix our hearts upon his religion, and bestow us with sincere penance, and that He complete us with goodness through His grace and His generosity.

CHAPTER THREE

MARTYRDOM AND THE PLAGUE

3.1

The Plague Is a Martyrdom and a Mercy for Muslims

THE CONTEXT SURROUNDING THE HADITHS THAT ATTEST TO THIS

Earlier we discussed Anas's hadith that states, "The plague is a martyrdom for all Muslims," and that its authenticity is agreed upon. We have also discussed the hadith of ʿĀʾisha that states that the plague is a "mercy" for the believers.[1] Another version of the same hadith, transmitted by Aḥmad ibn Ḥanbal, contains the phrase: "The ones who patiently endure the plague are like martyrs." In another version, Abū Yaʿlā had yet another phrasing: "Whoever is struck with the plague is a martyr." In the fourth chapter, we will discuss the hadith of Sharaḥbīl ibn Ḥasana that states: "Indeed, this plague is a mercy from your Lord."[2] Muʿādh's version has: "God awards the distinction of martyrdom to anyone among you that He wills."

God's Messenger said:

> "You all will go forth to Damascus, and it will be conquered. There will be a disease spread among you that is similar to that which causes abscesses or pain in one's heart, taking hold of man's abdomen.[3] God will make martyrs of them through it and purify their deeds through it."[4]

MARTYRDOM IS NOT ONLY FOR THOSE KILLED IN BATTLE

God's Messenger said:

> "Martyrs are of five kinds: one who dies of the plague, stomach ailment, drowning, a building collapse, and as a martyr fighting in the path of God."[5]

God's Messenger also said:

> "Who among you would be considered a martyr?"
>
> "Oh, God's Messenger! The one who dies fighting in the path of God—he is a martyr."
>
> "Then the martyrs of my community would be few."
>
> "So who are the martyrs, Prophet of God?"
>
> "Whoever is killed fighting in the path of God, he is a martyr. Whoever dies in the path of God, he is a martyr. Whoever dies from the plague, he is a martyr. Whoever dies from an ailment in his stomach, he is a martyr. The one who dies of drowning is a martyr."[6]

According to ʿĀʾisha, God's Messenger said:

> "The one who dies suffering from plague, from pleurisy, soon after childbirth, and from a stomach illness is a martyr."[7]

Saʿd said the Prophet said:

> "The fallen are granted martyrdom if they fell while fighting, suffering the plague, drowning, suffering from a stomach illness, while pregnant, and soon after giving childbirth."[8]

HADITHS ATTESTING TO OTHER KINDS OF MARTYRS

Consider this hadith, recorded in Mālik's *Well-Trodden Path*:

> When ʿAbdullāh ibn Thābit was in the throes of death, his daughter cried out, "By God! I hope you will become a martyr—for you have completed your preparation for battle."
>
> "God rewards according to one's intention," the Prophet replied. "Who among you do you consider to be a martyr?"
>
> "Those who died fighting in the path of God."
>
> "There are seven kinds of martyrdom other than dying fighting in the path of God: Someone killed by the plague is a martyr, someone drowned is a martyr, someone killed by pleurisy is a martyr, someone who dies of stomach illness is a martyr, someone who dies of a fire is a martyr, someone who dies in a building collapse, and a woman who dies while pregnant is a martyr."[9]

A text from ʿUbāda ibn al-Ṣāmit attests Mālik's narration of this hadith, but instead of "pleurisy," it lists "consumption"; instead of "a woman who dies pregnant," it has "death soon after childbirth; her child pulls her into heaven through his umbilical cord"; all of which has a similar meaning. In it, the Prophet also said: "The plague is a martyrdom"; but he does not mention "death by building collapse."[10]

The Prophet said:

> "Whoever falls off a mountaintop, whoever is eaten by a wild beast, and whoever drowns in the ocean will be martyrs in the eyes of God."[11]

The Prophet said:

> "The one experiencing seasickness at sea and vomits will have the reward of a martyr."[12]

The Prophet said:

> "Whoever is killed defending his wealth is a martyr."[13]

The Prophet said:

> "Whoever's neck is broken by his ass or his horse, or dies of an animal bite or a sting in the head, or dies on his bed mat while out in the path of God, then he is a martyr."[14]

The Prophet said:

> "Whoever dies stationed at a border fort dies a martyr."[15]

God's Messenger said:

> "The one who dies on his bed mat terrified, while out in the path of God, is a martyr . . . as is the one who dies of stomach pain, being bitten or stung, drowned, choked, killed by a wild beast, or tossed off his riding animal."[16]

God's Messenger said:

> "One who passes while abroad is a martyr."

Ibn ʿAbbās is cited as the source, but Ibn Mājah recorded it with a flimsy isnad. Al-Mundhirī said that martyrdom for one who dies abroad appears in a number of hadiths, but none of their isnads would be considered fair in terms of its reliability—that is what he said.

God's Messenger said:

> "Whoever falls in love but remains silent and holds back dies a martyr."[17]

The Prophet said:

> "Whoever recites the following when he wakes up: 'I seek refuge in God—all-seeing and all-knowing—from the accursed

> Devil,' and recites the last three verses from the Chapter of Assembly from the Qur'an, God assigns to him seventy thousand guardian angels who bless him until sunset. If he were to die that day, he would die a martyr. Whoever recites those things when he goes to sleep will have the same standing."[18]

The person who dies the kinds of deaths mentioned in these hadiths is a martyr, meaning that he will be given the reward of a martyr. Since most of these deaths are distressing, God bestowed benefits upon the community of Muhammad through them, making them a purification for their sins, and increasing their reward in paradise, even though, at the surface level, there are differences between them—but God knows best.

3.2

Martyrdom Is Obtained by Intention

The following hadiths are cited as evidence that, even if nothing like the things mentioned above strike the believer, martyrdom can still be obtained by intention alone. The Prophet said:

> "Whoever seeks martyrdom with sincerity, God will award it to him even if he does not reach his goal."[19]

Al-Ḥākim has another version of this hadith, which explains the one above:

> "Whoever sincerely asks God that he die in God's path, and then dies, God gives him the martyr's reward."[20]

The Prophet said:

> "Whoever sincerely asks God for martyrdom, God places him at the level of the martyrs, even if he dies in his bed."[21]

God's Messenger said:

> "Most of the martyrs of my community die in bed, but God knows best the intention of the many killed between the battle lines."[22]

Faḍāla ibn ʿUbayd said:

> Two men went out on a raid. One of them was slain in battle while the other died naturally. So Faḍāla sat at the grave of the one who died naturally, and he was told as much. He said: "I care little about which of the two graves I have sat myself beside." Then he recited the Qur'anic verse "Those who left their homes in the path of God and were slain or died, God will bless them with a handsome provision."[23]

Martyrdom was mentioned in Abū ʿInaba al-Khawlānī's presence.[24] He said that Muhammad's Companions told him that the Prophet spoke these words:

> "The martyrs of God on earth are trustees of God upon His creation, whether they are slain in battle or they die naturally."[25]

God's Messenger said:

> "God has his servants whom he keeps away from battle, lengthening their lives, giving them a good amount of wealth, and granting them long life in good health, taking their souls without affliction, resurrecting them without trials, and placing them on par with the martyrs."[26]

The point of these hadiths is to teach that martyrdom is divided into categories. First is the one considered a martyr in this world as well as in the hereafter—such as the one who is killed at war with the unbelievers, striving to elevate God's word. Second is one who is considered a martyr in this world alone—such as the one who is killed in a war with the unbelievers but did so while having corrupt intentions or while fleeing from the battle. The last is the one considered a martyr in the hereafter alone—one who is just that—but God knows best.

3.3
The Meaning of Martyr

The Arabic word for martyr—which literally means "witness"—is named that way, according to Ibn al-Anbārī, because God and the angels testify on his behalf for heaven. Al-Naḍr ibn Shumayl said it is so named because the martyr is in reality still alive, as if his soul still sees—meaning it is present. It is also said that the martyr is called a "witness" in Arabic because he witnesses the honor God has reserved for him when his soul leaves his body. A fourth opinion is that it is because the only things he witnesses at his death are the angels of mercy. A fifth is that it is because the angels testify as to his excellent ending. A sixth opinion is that this is because the prophets testify as to the excellence of his following of their example. A seventh is that it is because God testifies as to the excellence of his intention and his sincerity. An eighth opinion is that it is based upon the testimony of the community of believers that he belongs in paradise. A ninth is that it is because he testifies that messengers conveyed their message on the Day of Judgment. A tenth opinion is that it is because he witnesses the angels at the moment of his demise. An eleventh is that it is because he witnesses two realms simultaneously: this world and the hereafter. A twelfth opinion is that it is because he is witnessed as saved from the fires of hell. Lastly, it is said that it is so named because he has a mark that testifies that he has attained salvation.

Some of these opinions only apply to the martyr on the battlefield, and some of them could be applied to that as well as others. Some of them include what relates to both the unmartyred and the martyred.

THE SPECIAL CHARACTERISTICS OF THE MARTYR IN THE AFTERLIFE

The Prophet said:

> "God's martyr will have six things waiting for him: He will be forgiven the instant his blood is spilt and he will see his seat in paradise; he will be protected from the torment of the grave; he will be saved from the Great Terror of the Day of Judgment;* upon his head will be placed the crown of dignity; and he will be married to seventy-two heavenly nymphs; and on the Day of Judgment, he will intercede for seventy of his close relatives."[27]

Martyrs are actually alive in the presence of their Lord, who provides them with sustenance, as has been established in a proof-text from the Qur'an. In al-Bukhārī's *Authentic Hadith*, it is established that the souls of the martyrs are "inside bountiful and verdant green birds flying freely in paradise, who then roost in lanterns hanging from the Throne of God."

The attributes of a martyr include the characteristic that he wishes he could return to the life of this world because he saw the honor and the merit of his martyrdom, as has been established in al-Bukhārī's *Authentic Hadith*. Another one of the martyr's attributes is that paradise is apportioned for him, regardless of his sins—we already previously discussed our research on the duties he owes to other human beings.

---

*A reference to Qur'an 21:103: "The Great Terror [of the Day of Judgment] shall not grieve them, and the angels will welcome them, saying, 'This is your Day that you have been promised.'"

3.4
Praying for Martyrdom

What is the answer to those who object that praying for martyrdom requires empowering an unbeliever to kill a believer, which is a sinful act, and therefore appears to contradict the principle that prohibits wishing for a sin against God?

The essence of the reply is this: The goal that is sought is only obtaining elevated status. As for the unbeliever's act, it is only out of necessity that it must be. It is on this view that the desire for death is understood for those who wished for martyrdom among the greats of the Companions of the Prophet and others. Similarly, this is the view that justifies wishing for death from the plague, as in the case of the Companion Muʿādh ibn Jabal and others.

ʿUmar wished for martyrdom, and when the Persian slave Abū Luʾluʾa killed him, it was taken as a good omen because his assassin was an unbeliever. The most sublime saying concerning this matter is the saying of the Prophet:

"I wish that I were killed in the path of God, then brought back to life so I could be killed again."[28]

3.5
Hadiths That Prove That Some Martyrs Are Superior to Others

God's Messenger said:

> "Death on the battlefield is of three kinds:
>
> The first is a person who struggles in the path of God with his person and his wealth to the point that when he meets the

enemy, he fights to his own death. That is the proud martyr in the tent of the Almighty and Exalted God, and dignified under God's Throne. Even the prophets would not be superior to him were it not for their status of prophethood.

The second is a believer who loathes himself on account of his sins and errors. He struggles in the path of God with his person and his wealth to the point that, when he likewise meets the enemy, he fights to his own death. In doing so, he wipes away his moral shortcomings, for the sword is the effacer of errors. He enters through any gate to paradise he wishes—for heaven has eighty gates, and some are superior to others.

Lastly, the dissembling hypocrite who struggles with his person and his wealth, to the point that when he meets the enemy he fights to his own death. He is sent to the fires of hell, for the sword does not efface hypocrisy."[29]

Consider this hadith as well:

A man came to God's Messenger while he was praying. Then that man turned to the row of worshippers when he finished:

"O God, give me things more excellent than what you give your righteous servants."

"Who spoke those words?" the Prophet asked when he finished his prayer.

"I did, Prophet of God!"

"Your steed will be wounded in battle, and you will become a martyr in the path of God."[30]

Consider this hadith as well:

A man asked God's Messenger: "Which kind of martyr is best?"

"Those who, when thrown into a battle line, do not swerve their faces until they are killed. Those are the martyrs who will see the highest levels of paradise, and your Lord will beam with joy upon them. Once your Lord smiles upon a servant, there is no reckoning in store for him."[31]

Finally, there is the story of the man whom the Antichrist killed, about whom the Prophet said:

> "In terms of martyrdom, he will be the greatest of the people in the eyes of the Lord of the worlds."[32]

3.6

A Martyr of the Plague Is Like a Martyr on the Battlefield

Even though it is true that those who die on the battlefield share in martyrdom with those who die of the plague, there are many aspects in which these groups are not treated equally. For example, unlike those martyred by the plague, the religious laws prescribe that the bodies of those martyred on the battlefield are not enshrouded or washed, and that funeral prayers are not said for them. Moreover, the bodies of those martyred by war will not be afflicted in the grave, and they are actually alive in the presence of their Lord and provided sustenance by Him—a distinction not shared by martyrs of the plague. However, those believers who die of the plague do share in the rewards of martyrdom alongside the martyrs of war, and they share some aspects related to the afterlife.

The Prophet said:

> "The martyrs and those who die of the plague will come forward on the Day of Judgment. Those who died of the plague will say: 'We are martyrs.' Someone will call out: 'Examine them! If their wounds are like the wounds of martyrs flowing with blood, and their scent is like the scent of musk, then they are martyrs.' They will then find their blood and scent to be just so."[33]

God's Messenger also said:

> "The martyrs and those who die naturally on their beds will take their dispute on the status of those who died from the plague to our Lord, lofty in His highness. The martyrs will assert that 'our brothers who died of the plague were killed just like we were killed in battle.' Those who died naturally on their beds will argue that 'our brothers who died of the plague passed away on their beds like we passed away.' God Almighty and Exalted will respond: 'Examine their wounds. If they resemble the wounds of those killed in battle, then they are martyrs.' And lo and behold: their wounds will resemble the wounds of the martyrs of the battlefield."[34]

This hadith was also recorded by al-Kalābādhī. In the text of that variant of the hadith, the Prophet said:

> "God settled the dispute between them, saying: 'Examine the wounds of those pierced by plague. If they resemble the wounds of the martyrs on the battlefield, then they are martyrs.' So they examined the wounds of those pierced by plague, and they did indeed resemble the wounds of the martyrs on the battlefield. Thus, they attain the same status."[35]

3.7

Criteria for Meriting Martyrdom by Plague

ʿĀʾisha said:

> I once asked the Messenger of God about the plague. He told me: "The plague was a torment sent by God upon anyone He wills, but which He makes a mercy upon the believers.

> There is not a man whom the plague strikes that does not receive the bounty of martyrdom—as long as he remains in his home in patience and hopeful for heavenly reward, knowing that it shall not strike him unless God has already inscribed such a fate for him, and unless God apportioned him the martyr's reward."[36]

Both the letter and spirit of this hadith necessitate that the reward of the martyr is inscribed for anyone who does not flee the place in which the plague occurs. It also requires that he intend in his patience to obtain God's reward, having full hope in the truth of His promised bounty. It also requires that he knows that God predetermines whether the plague strikes him or passes over him. That means that he must not be discontent with God if the plague strikes him. Rather, if the plague strikes him, then he should be content and rely on his Lord for his health and recovery. To this end, whoever embodies these character traits and then dies of something other than the plague, then it is apparent from the hadith that the reward of a martyr is granted for him.

It must be emphasized, in our view, that the degrees of martyrdom vary. Dying patiently at home of something other than the plague, during a plague, is like someone who goes off to war from his home intending to struggle in God's way on the battlefield, and then dies afterward of something other than battle. This is supported by the previous narration of the hadith of Abū Hurayra with the phrasing "Whoever dies during the plague is a martyr."[37] He deliberately did not phrase it "Whoever dies *by* the plague," so its apparent meaning is as a testament to what we asserted above.

If one were to construe the phrase "during the plague" to mean "because of the plague" to exclude those who did not die because of it, then consider that the literal wording of the same hadith states: "Whosoever dies in the stomach is a martyr." It is well-known that the intended meaning here refers to the person who dies of the stomach ailment itself. It is also possible to construe the word "during" as a grammatical term that indicates circumstantial conditions, with the caveat that "it" refers to the predominant circumstances, while understanding that death during the plague is mostly because of those circumstances. The final possibility is to interpret the phrase "during the plague" in the circumstantial sense and the causal sense at the same time.

This raises the question: If a person has the character traits of a martyr, and yet the plague goes away and he does not die by it—nor does he die even during the time of the plague—is that person a martyr or not?

The apparent sense of the hadith covers his case, as the bounty of God is wide, and the intention of the believer is more effective than his acts. The prophetic hadith from Ibn Masʿūd we just saw refers to this: "Most of the martyrs of my community die in bed." Similarly, we can also cite the hadith from Jābir ibn ʿAtīk, in which the Prophet said: "God grants reward commensurate with intention."

Al-Subkī said:

> The lesson we can take from the meaning of the hadith is that the believer's intention is more effective than his actions. This is because the extent of one's intention has no limitations, while one's actions are restricted. The value of one's intentions is commensurate with what it is connected to, which can be great or small.

Do not be led into the following confusion: that whosoever has the character traits of a martyr, then dies of the plague, must be granted the reward of two martyrdoms. We removed any such confusion with what we discussed previously—that degrees of martyrdom vary—so the degree of martyrdom is elevated for anyone who is characterized by those traits and then is pierced by the plague and dies of it. Lower in status to him is the one who exemplifies the character traits of a martyr and then is pierced by the plague but does not die of it. Near to him in status is he who has the character but is not pierced by the plague and does not die of it.

The reward for martyrdom may multiply when the causes upon which the levels of martyrdom depend are differentiated.

For instance, consider how different the status would be of someone who were to die abroad of the plague, with patience and hoping for heavenly reward. Or how different the status would be of a woman who was struck by plague during labor but then died in childbirth. This would hold as well for any of the sayings or actions we discussed previously that lead to martyrdom.

Another issue is raised concerning this possibility: the proliferation of the number of portions of heavenly reward for the one who participates in multiple funeral prayers.[38] Similarly, a group of the Prophet's Companions related that whosoever acquires dogs will have their heavenly reward decrease in proportion to the number of dogs. Indeed, if one accepts that heavenly rewards proliferate in the case of funeral prayers, then it is more so the case in different types of martyrdom, because God multiplies the reward for good deeds, but does not multiply the punishment for sin.

It is possible to say that the rank of martyrdom is one thing, while the rewards of martyrdom are another. Martyrdom is therefore distinguished first by the aforementioned character traits, and then it is distinguished further if one is pierced by the plague and dies of it.

Then I saw this very same view in the words of Ibn Abī Jamra in a commentary on a section from al-Bukhārī's *Authentic Hadith*, which he summarized. In his discourse on this hadith, he discussed the difference between the two narrations. It says in the preceding hadith that "the one pierced by the plague is a martyr" and that "to him it is a reward *akin* to the martyr." On this view, whoever does not fit the description of a martyr of this type obtains the reward of the martyr, even if he does not obtain the status of the martyr.

One implication drawn from ʿĀʾisha's hadith is that anyone who does not have the character traits of a martyr does not become a martyr even if he dies of the plague, to say nothing of other kinds of death—may God help us.

Another conclusion drawn from ʿĀʾisha's hadith is that the one who is patient during the plague, exemplifying the character traits of a martyr, will be safe from the trials of the grave because he is comparable to the one who mans the border forts for the sake of jihad in God's path. As Salmān heard the Messenger of God say:

> "Keeping guard for a day and a night is better than fasting and observing the night prayers for a month. If one dies while keeping guard, he goes to his death while doing that good act—and in this way, he is saved from the trials of the grave."[39]

The Messenger of God also said:

> "The fate of everyone who dies is sealed upon their final act except the one who keeps guard. His final act advances him to the Day of Resurrection, and he is saved from the trials of the grave."[40]

Abū Yaʿlā recorded this version of the hadith:

> "Whoever fights and perseveres until he is killed or victorious, he is safeguarded from the trial of the grave."[41]

3.8

Plague Is a Martyrdom and a Mercy

THE ANSWERS TO THE OBJECTIONS THAT ARISE CONCERNING THIS ISSUE

God's Messenger said:

> "Along the mountain-paths to Medina there are angels, such that neither the plague nor the Antichrist can gain entrance there."[42]

God's Messenger said:

> "The Antichrist will approach Medina but find angels there. Thus, neither the Antichrist nor the plague can gain entrance there, if God wills, may He be exalted."[43]

The objection is then raised: If the plague is both a martyrdom and a mercy, how is it connected with the Antichrist? And how is the noble city of Medina commended by the fact that the plague does not gain entrance there?

The answer to this question is the following: The occurrence of the plague is indeed a martyrdom and a mercy, but that characterization is not intended to describe the plague itself. Rather, it means that martyrdom and mercy result from it, arise from it, and are caused by it. If you accept that, and you call to mind the preceding chapter on the phrase "the pricks of the jinn," it becomes apparent that this hadith lauds Medina by the fact that the plague does not enter it, signaling that the unbelievers among the jinn and their demons are forbidden from entering the noble city of Medina. And whoever among the jinn happens to enter it will not be able to pierce any of its people, as God offers them protection from the jinn.

As the evidence demonstrated earlier, the piercing of the jinn is not limited to the unbelievers among the jinn striking the believers of humankind, rather, the piercing is exacted by believers among the jinn upon the unbelievers of humankind. Therefore, even if it is accepted that the unbelieving jinn are prevented from entering Medina, how can it be that the believers among the jinn are prevented from entering?

The answer is the following: The entry of unbelievers into Medina is not permissible, therefore no one resides in Medina except those who outwardly live by Islam; the laws of the Muslims are applied to them, such that even one who is not sincere in his Islam follows the one who is sincere, so in that way they obtain protection from the arrival of the jinn. That is why the plague does not enter the city at all.

This answer is better than the one given by al-Qurṭubī in

The Discerning, where he argues that "the meaning of the hadith is that no plague enters Medina that is comparable in severity to others, such as the Plague of ʿAmwās and the Plague of al-Jārif." It is a fitting answer upon confirmation of the descent of the plague upon Medina if anything like that were to ever occur in it.[44]

Others said that the reason the plague does not enter Medina is that God's mercy is not limited simply to the plague. The Prophet prayed to God, noting, "But your granting of good health is easier for me." Thus, good health is one of the special characteristics of the noble city of Medina. The Prophet continuously prayed to God for the city's good health. This is the essence of what al-Millawī and al-Subkī argued.

A number of other answers were offered by al-Manbijī. Among them, he suggested that the fact that the plague does not enter Medina is a miracle. From the first physicians to the last, none have been capable of repelling the plague from a single city or even a single village. Yet, for this continuous duration, the plague has been prevented from entering Medina due to the Prophet's prayer and by his knowledge from God to that effect. But this is not, in my opinion, an answer to the objection raised at the beginning of this chapter.

Another answer he offered was what was previously discussed—that Medina is protected from the demons who strike the believers with plague.

In another reply to the objections, he argued that the Prophet exchanged the plague for fever, because the plague comes from time to time, whereas the fever recurs in every era, so they balance out. Alternatively, he suggested that the fact that the plague would not enter Medina was unique to the time of the Prophet. Yet another explanation for why the Prophet exchanged the plague for fever was that Medina is such a small city; if the plague ever did occur there, the totality of its inhabitants would perish.

It is apparent to me that there is an answer more particular than these various solutions—after calling to mind when God's Messenger said: "Gabriel came to me offering either fever or the plague, so I seized on the choice of fever for Medina, and sent the plague to Damascus. . . ."[45] The answer to the objection, based on this hadith, is that there is wisdom in sending the plague to Damascus and keeping the fever for Medina. When the Prophet entered Medina, there were few of his Companions in number and few reinforcements and provisions and other things, and Medina was stricken by a pestilence, as was demonstrated previously by the hadith of ʿĀʾisha. Thus, his prayer for Medina's health, for the recovery of its inhabitants so they may engage in jihad against the unbelievers was consistent with the context. The Prophet was made to choose between the two diseases—the fever and the plague—and anyone who would have been struck by either of them would receive a magnificent heavenly reward. He selected, at that time, the fever for Medina, because its burden was lighter than the plague's, on account of the typical speed of the plague's mortality. Then, when the Prophet was permitted to take up fighting, it continued to be a problem that the fever was weakening the bodies that needed strength in the jihad. So, at that time, he asked God to move the fever to al-Juḥfa, and his prayers were answered. And then Medina became the healthiest of the cities of God, may He be exalted.

So when God willed death to any of them by fever, that person would receive the martyrdom that was in store for those who died by the plague, and for those killed fighting in the path of God, which is the highest level of martyrdom. This was true for anyone who died of the kind of fever that relieves the believer from the fire, as every day of fever is a year's worth of atonement. And it continued that way in Medina after the time of the Prophet, and it distinguishes that city from all other cities, as a realization of the answer to the Prophet's prayers.

Of course, the noble city of Mecca shares in that protection with Medina, as no plague has entered that city over the passage of time, as Ibn Qutayba asserted in *The Knowledge*, and most of the learned scholars repeated that and confirmed it, up to the time of al-Nawawī, who repeated it in his *Book of Remembrances* and other places.

However, it is said that, after that, it did enter Mecca during the Great Plague, which occurred in the year 749 (1348), and again after that. If that were shown to be true, perhaps it is because its sacred space was violated by unbelievers living there, particularly during our own time, and then it was put to a halt. Only God can help us.

3.9

The Response to Another Objection to the Claim That the Plague Is a Martyrdom and a Mercy

God's Messenger approached us and said:

> "Behold, community of emigrants! There are five afflictions by which you will be tested—and I seek refuge in God lest you live to see them: When moral indecency appears among a people and they commit it openly, plagues and sicknesses that their predecessors never suffered will spread among them. When they manipulate the measures and scales of the marketplace, they will be seized by famine, hardship, and the ruler's injustice upon them. When they withhold zakat on their wealth, they are denied rain from the skies; and were it not for the animals, it would not rain at all. When they break the covenant with God or his Messenger, God imposes the rule of their foreign enemies upon them, who will seize some of their wealth. When their leaders fail to rule by the book of God and fail to seek goodness only in what God has revealed, God will cause conflict among them."[46]

In Ibn ʿAbbās's version, God's Messenger said:

> "When deception appears among a people, God delivers terror to their hearts. When fornication spreads among a

people, death certainly multiplies among them. When a people manipulate the scales and measures of the marketplace, their sustenance will be cut off. When the people rule by other than the truth, bloodshed becomes widespread among them. When the people break covenants, their enemies are empowered over them."[47]

In ʿAmr ibn al-ʿĀṣ's version, God's Messenger said:

> "When fornication appears among a people, they are seized with annihilation. When usury appears among a people, they are seized by drought. When bribery appears among a people, they are seized by terror."[48]

In Abū ʿAbdullāh ibn Burayda's version, God's Messenger said:

> "When a people fail to satisfy their covenants in any way, there will be fighting among them. When moral indecency appears in the people in any way, God imposes death upon them. When the people refrain from paying zakat, God withholds even a drop of rain from them."[49]

Ibn ʿAbbās also said God's Messenger said:

> "When illegitimate children and usury appear in a community, they have made themselves liable to the wrath of God, may He be exalted."[50]

Maymūna said God's Messenger said:

> "My community will continue to be blessed, as long as illegitimate children do not become prevalent among them. But if illegitimate children become prevalent among them, God will be quick to encompass them in punishment."[51]

The contradiction that emerges from these hadiths is the following: How can the plague be a martyrdom and a mercy, when the full thrust of these hadiths necessitates that God—may He be exalted—delivered the plague as a punishment for the perpetration of sin?

The answer is the following: There is no contradiction between them. It is part of God's mercy for this Muhammadan community that He hastens for them their punishments in this world. For in a hadith, God's Messenger said:

> "My community is a community granted mercy; there is no punishment for it in the hereafter—its punishment in this life is civil strife, earthquakes, and war."[52]

God's Messenger said:

> "My community is holy, blessed, and granted mercy. There is to be no punishment for my community on the Day of Resurrection. Rather, my community endures punishment in this world."[53]

God's Messenger said:

> "The punishment of this community is by the sword."[54]

Mālik al-Ashjaʿī said:

> Abū Hurayra said: "God's Messenger said: 'This community is a community granted mercy. There is no punishment upon it other than the punishment it inflicts on itself.'"
>
> Abū Ḥāzim asked Abū Hurayra, "How would the community punish itself?"
>
> Abū Hurayra replied: "Was not the Battle of Nahar a punishment? Was not the Battle of the Camel a torment? Was not the Battle of Ṣiffīn* a punishment?"[55]

---

*These three battles were bitter watershed events during the partisan civil wars over succession and power following Muhammad's death and the deaths of his earliest successors.

In my view, the above hadith explains the meaning of Abū Mūsā's hadith that the community's "punishment in this world is civil strife, earthquakes, and war." It is a strong corroborating version for it, and it cannot be said to be Abū Hurayra's personal opinion. It ought to be construed as applying to the majority of the community of Muhammad, as has been established by the hadith on intercession that there will be people of Muhammad's community that "are punished, then rescued from the fire and admitted to paradise."

However, the intent of the hadith—that the plague is a punishment from God on account of a violation of His commandments—does not contradict the fact that its occurrence is also a martyrdom and a mercy in the case of all believers whom it pierces. This is the case especially because most of the believers have not committed the abominations mentioned above. However, perhaps the punishment applies to all of them because they refrained from commanding right and forbidding wrong or because they abandoned giving pious advice to others. Alternatively, it could be because those who are upright sullied themselves with the kinds of sins that are less than abominations, so their words are no longer heeded and their lectures are not accepted. There is no might nor power except with God Almighty, the Most High.

The intent of the hadith could be to increase the good deeds of one who does not commit acts of moral indecency, who is not lax in the duty to command the right and forbid the wrong. This has been established in another hadith from Abū Hurayra, who said that God's Messenger said:

> "In the hereafter, it could be the case that a person has a high station in God's eyes, and yet does not make it to that level with his deeds alone. So God continues to afflict that person with things he abhors until he reaches it."[56]

Now, that was the answer for those for whom the plague is a martyrdom and a mercy, in contrast to those for whom it is not; in that case, the plague is nothing except a pure punishment. Thus, you find many kinds of people to whom the latter applies. Being struck by the plague intensifies such a person's unease and magnifies his discontent and disgust. Such a person tries to outwit the disease in many ways. He repels it with a variety of things that are said to do so: incantations, rings, incenses, amulets that are worn over one's head, and writing on one's doors. He gets involved in all manner of fortune-telling, which the religious law forbids, and avoids many foods and things like that. He assigns the disease's cause to the wind and the water, without looking into its real cause and its true substance. He avoids funerals, even though it would soften his heart, draw his tears, humble him, and make him fear God. He also dallies in other corrupt things that would forbid him a heavenly reward and martyrdom similar to that which is attained through patience and self-reflection.

Most of these corrupted people die of something other than the plague during the time of plague, and so the status of martyrdom slips away from them, and they go out of this world unwillingly. However, anyone who concludes their life by dying as a Muslim has attained salvation from the everlasting hellfire. The hadith report at the beginning of this chapter confirms this, since one of the clearest causes of the plague is the proliferation of fornication, as was discussed previously at the end of the first chapter, regarding the story of Balaam and Moses—but God knows best.

In fact, we find many righteous people who stand in contrast to the attributes above. They are divided into several grades:

There are those who go to their death joyfully, as did the pious predecessors, such as Muʿādh ibn Jabal and others. There are those who go to their death surrendering to God, trusting and accepting of God's will, even though they do not love that they are dying, as is anyone's natural disposition. There are also those who go to their death overly preoccupied with themselves, afraid of death striking them before they can clear themselves of the duties they owe to others. So, for those kinds of people, we beg God's pardon and forgiveness through His grace and His generosity.

It is clear to me that the fact that moral indecency is a cause of the plague—if that report is authentic—contains a response to the description of the jinn as "brothers of humankind"—that is, that the jinn are "brothers in religion." The response it contains is the following: the penalty for premarital sex is flogging, while the penalty for extramarital sex is to be put to death in a particular way.[57] It is not far-fetched to think that the believers among the jinn are given authority over humankind to apply the punishment against the fornicator by piercing him with the plague, practically executing whoever committed extramarital sex, and likewise to torment whoever committed the lesser sin of premarital sex. Or they may strike humankind in a form of warfare because of the emergence of moral indecency among them and their neglect of the duty to censure that. When a war is waged, the casualties occur among everyone; the killed are simply brought back to life on the Day of Resurrection, according to the sincerity of their intention. This has been established by the hadith containing the story of the army that the earth swallowed up, as Muslim and Abū Dāwūd recorded from the hadith of Umm Salama. As the Prophet's wife, Umm Salama, recalled, the Prophet said:

> "When sins appear in my community, God will punish everyone who has committed them."
>
> "Messenger of God!" I said. "What about the righteous ones among them?"
>
> "Yes, they will be struck by what strikes the general populace. Then they will be forgiven and accepted by God."[58]

ʿĀʾisha said the Prophet said:

> "Then God will bring them back from the dead according to the sincerity of their intention."[59]

These hadiths are the best clarification that there is no contradiction between calling the plague a "punishment" and a "mercy," as long as each of the two descriptions is read in light of the other.

There is nothing preventing God from permitting the believers among the jinn to punish anyone He wishes among humankind by the plague, even if there are those who have not sinned among them, just as He has given permission to some of the angels to make the ground swallow up a village in which there are some innocent people, or sink a great ship, or inflict a tremendous earthquake that destroys many homes in which many people die in the destruction. Afterward, their homes in the hereafter will be quite different. Disobedience is not ascribed to those angels who undertake those acts, nor is it ascribed to the believers among the jinn. Rather, the correct description of jinn is as brothers, brothers in faith. As for the occurrence of the "enemies" phrase in some hadiths, we have covered that already—but God knows best.

I later found the source of this reply to the objection described in the same volume of al-Manbijī I mentioned earlier. He phrased it in this way:

> It is possible that the believers among the jinn are given power over the people who commit acts of immorality, such as extramarital sex and other cases in which it is lawful to execute people. But the believer among the jinn is not permitted to kill the believer of humankind purposefully if he does not have grounds for doing so.

Some of this was suggested previously in the words of Ibn al-Qayyim in the second chapter—but God knows best.

CHAPTER FOUR

AGAINST FLIGHT FROM THE PLAGUE

4.1

Evidence for the Prohibition of Fleeing the Plague

God, the Glorified, the Exalted, said:

> Have you not seen those who fled their homes, fearing death, by the thousands? God commanded them, "Die!" but then brought them back to life.[1]

ʿAbd al-Razzāq noted a report on this verse in his *Exegesis of the Qur'an*; he said:

> They fled from the plague, so God commanded them to die, but then brought them back to life to live out the remainder of their lives.[2]

Ibn Abī Ḥātim recorded this report:

> When the plague occurred, one third escaped, but two-thirds stayed. Then the plague struck again, and another two-thirds fled, and a third remained. Then the plague struck again, and the rest left hastily. Then God made them die as a punishment.[3]

Al-Ṭabarī recorded this report:

> They left fleeing from the plague, and God caused them to die before their appointed time. Then he resurrected them to live out the rest of their lives.[4]

ʿAbd ibn Ḥamīd notes the following report in his *Exegesis of the Qur'an*:

> God loathed them for fleeing from death, so he caused them to die as a punishment, then resurrected them to live out the rest of their lives, so that they may again die. If they reached their appointed times of death, they would not have been resurrected.[5]

Ibn Abī Ḥātim recorded a long story commenting on the Qur'anic verse that opened this chapter:

> There was a village close to Wāsiṭ called Dāwardān. The plague struck the people who lived there. One group of them stayed, and the other fled, abandoning it completely. The plague struck those who stayed and spread through them quickly, while those who fled were untouched. When the plague was lifted from them, the party who fled returned. Those who stayed said to themselves: "Our brothers were more decisive than us. If we had had done as they did, we would have been safe. If only we had stayed just until the plague started and done as they did."
>
> After some time, the plague reoccurred, and this time everyone fled—both those who abandoned the village the last time and those who stayed, numbering a little more than thirty thousand. They wandered until they reached an expansive valley between two mountains and settled there.
>
> Then God sent two angels to them, one angel from the high end of the valley and the other from its lowest point. The angels announced the command for them to die and to remain dead for as long as God willed. So they died.
>
> Then, one day, a prophet named Ezekiel passed by them and saw all the bones. He stopped, struck in amazement at their sheer number. God inspired him to announce: "Bones: God commands you to assemble!" All the bones, from the farthest part of the valley to its lowest part, came together, some of them reattached to others. Each bone from a given body came together to form the frame of that particular body. They became fully formed skeletons but without flesh or blood. Then God inspired him to announce, "Bones:

> God commands you to clothe yourself in flesh!" and they clothed themselves with flesh. And then God inspired him to announce, "Bodies: God commands you to stand up!" Lo and behold—they were resurrected, alive!
>
> Then they returned to their lands. The only clothing they had were their shrouds, which served as their tribal marker, and by which people recognized them as belonging to those of that era. They lived, afterward, for as long as their appointed times.[6]

Al-Ṭabarī records another long version of this hadith. The following passage exists in that version:

> When he saw them, he halted in his tracks. When he started to think about them, he frowned and curled his fingers. God spoke to him: "Ezekiel, do you want me to show you how I resurrect them?" He replied, "Yes." He could not stop wondering at God's power over them.[7]

Al-Ṭabarī also preserved the following addition:

> When they returned to their people alive, their people recognized that they had been dead because of the look of death on their faces.

Al-Ṭabarī and Ibn Abī Ḥātim recorded another long version of this hadith. This version does not name the prophet mentioned nor provide a number for the dead. Moreover, those who left said: "Had we stayed as those who did, we would have perished as they perished." The ones who stayed said: "Had we fled as those who fled, we would have been saved as they were saved." In this version, the prophet passes by them and says:

> "Lord! Had you willed to allow them to live, they would have lived a long life in Your lands and worshipped You."
>
> God asked: "Is that what you want me to do?"

"Yes," said the prophet.

God commanded him: "Then utter the following words . . ."

The prophet spoke those words as he looked at the bones. The different bones gathered themselves to the bodies to which they belonged. Then he gave another command, and suddenly the bones were covered with flesh. Then he gave another command, and they sat up in haste, praising and glorifying God. Then they were commanded, "Fight in God's path!"[8]

This report has another sound isnad through the Companion Ibn 'Abbās,[9] but the text is abbreviated:

They were four thousand in number and left fleeing from the plague. They said, "We will go to a place where death does not exist." Yet, when they reached a certain place, God commanded them, "Die!" Sometime later, a prophet walked past them and prayed to God to resurrect them, and God did so.[10]

A different perspective is conveyed in the following report, which cites Ash'ath ibn Aslam al-Baṣrī:

When 'Umar was praying, there were two Jews behind him. One of them said to other, "Is that him?"

When 'Umar turned around, he asked them what they wanted.

"We found you in God's book described as a rod of iron," they said. "You would be given what Ezekiel—who brought the dead back to life with God's permission—was given."

'Umar said, "We do not find anything about Ezekiel in God's book. No one brought the dead back to life with God's permission except Jesus."

"Do you not find the following verse in God's book? 'And messengers whom we have not narrated their stories to you . . .'"[11]

"I do."

"He was one of them. As for bringing the dead back to life, we will tell you the following story: When pestilence struck the Israelites, a group of them escaped. When they found themselves upon the top of a slope, God caused them to die. Afterward, the Israelites built a wall on top of them. When their bones had disintegrated, God sent Ezekiel, who stood over them and said, 'This is what God wills.' Then God resurrected them for him. God revealed the following verse about them: 'Have you not seen those who fled their homes, fearing death, by the thousands . . .'"[12]

While all of these narrations reinforce each other, there are others attributed to Ibn ʿAbbās that are unique. The first group of these unique narrations concerns the cause of their resurrection:

What is meant by the phrase "by the thousands" in the Qur'anic verse is simply a large number. They were commanded to fight in God's cause but fled from the jihad, and thus God caused them to die. Then He brought them back to life and commanded them to return to the jihad.[13]

The second group of these anomalous narrations concerns the period of time that elapsed between the deaths of the people and their being brought back to life. Al-Qurṭubī transmits a report that some said the period was seven days, others saying it was eight days, and some saying it was a month, and yet others saying it was more than a month. However, the apparent sense of the reports cited above required that it was more than all these possibilities, because their bodies and their fleshy sinews had decomposed and turned into bones.

Al-Ṭabarī records another report citing ʿAmr ibn Dīnār that explained the verse, "Have you not seen those who fled their homes, fearing death, by the thousands . . ." in the following way:

The plague took place in their village. Some of the people left, and others stayed. Of the ones who stayed, some perished

> and others lived. Then another plague occurred. The people who left this time were more than the ones who left the first time, but still some remained, and some of those perished. Then there was a third plague. All but a few left. God caused them to die and then brought them back to life. The resurrected returned to their old town, where the children of those who were left behind were now living. Each one would ask the other: "Who are you?"[14]

Ibn al-Mundhir records another version from Ibn ʿAbbās:

> When the plague occurred and the people fled, those left behind waited for those who fled, but they never returned. Those left behind rode out and found that those who fled were dead, but they were unable to bury them, so they fenced them in by erecting a wall. Then, after some time, God resurrected them, and there was not a single one who had lost even a turban cord, much less the scarf it holds in place.
>
> Afterward, they returned to their town.
>
> A man would head to his house and find his son and grandson or even his great-grandson and cry out, "This is my house!"
>
> "This isn't your house," his descendent would protest, "but mine and that of my father."
>
> "Who are you?" the one who had been resurrected would ask.
>
> "I am so and so, son of so and so, son of . . ." until his descendent listed the person he had just met![15]

The main point of this report is that it offers evidence of the length of time between their deaths and their being brought back to life. But God knows best.

The third group of anomalous narrations concerns the number of those who fled, died, and were resurrected. Most of the preceding narrations say they were four thousand.[16] Al-Thaʿlabī quotes al-Suddī as having the view that they were a little over thirty-one thousand. Al-Thaʿlabī and, subsequently, al-Qurṭubī claimed, "It was said that they were forty thousand, seventy thousand, eighty thousand, ninety thousand, or one hundred thousand."

Al-Ṭabarī, in his commentary on the phrase "by the thousands," held that the most correct view is that their number was more than ten thousand, as opposed to those who say it was lower than that, because the Arabic grammatical form used in the Qur'anic verse for "thousands" is a plural indicating abundance, which is not used for anything that is less than ten thousand; a different Arabic grammatical form would be used for that. One group of exegetes followed him on this issue.

Another group of expert scholars, however, responded that it is possible to apply the plural form indicating abundance used in the Qur'anic verse under discussion to less than a thousand. This is the case, for example, in the Qur'anic phrase for "three periods."[17] Moreover, when the situation requires conveying the meaning of abundance, this is explicitly indicated. In the case of the number of people who fled and died, the context of the story, in addition to the fact that the strongest isnad recorded in Ibn ʿAbbās's view is four thousand, clarifies their true number. Meanwhile, the isnads of all other views, with the exception of Ibn ʿAbbās's above, have some problems—especially al-Suddī's view that "they were a little over thirty-one thousand."

It is possible to reconcile the Ibn ʿAbbās and al-Suddī views: the lower number could refer just to the chiefs and elites, while the larger one includes their followers as well. But God knows best.

The fourth group of anomalous narrations concerns the fact that all of the narrations, regardless of whether they were strong or weak, agree that the meaning of the original Arabic phrase for "thousands"—ulūf—refers to a number. The exception is what al-Ṭabarī records from ʿAbd al-Raḥmān ibn Aslam, who offers the following interpretation of the Qur'anic phrase "in their thousands": "The word 'ulūf' does not refer to a group but rather to the fact that their hearts were brought together in fellowship as they fled." His view requires interpreting the word "ulūf" (fellows) as a plural of "ilf" (fellow, singular).[18] Al-Ṭabarī held that the majority, who define the term as a number, are most likely to be correct. Al-Zamakhsharī held that the view that defined the word "ulūf" as something other than a number was a heretical view in the field of Qur'anic exegesis.

Ibn ʿAṭiyya noted that:

> The stories of those who fled all have weak isnads, but their main point is God's causing a people who fled death to die and subsequently to be brought back to life. He did so to show the futility of the worrier's alarm and the fool's self-delusion.

Abū Bakr ibn al-ʿArabī said:

> The opinion that the phrase "by the thousands" actually means "in fellowship" is weak, because death occurred to them despite their great numbers, a fact that results in even greater reflection on their story. This is because the death of such a large number all at once is unusual, which amplifies their case as a great warning to humankind. As for God striking to death a people who are characterized by fellowship and love, this would be just as if it were visited upon a people characterized by animosity. It does nothing to change the effectiveness of the warning.

Fakhr al-Dīn al-Rāzī responded to the "fellowship" interpretation with the following:

> It is possible that the intent of the phrase in question is that each one of those fleeing was attached to his life and in love with this world, as opposed to being attached to those with whom he fled. The point then returns to what God said in the verse "You will find them the most eager in clinging to life."[19] Because of the extreme amount of love for this worldly life and their attachment to it, God caused them to die, so that they might know that their greed for this life will not protect them from death.

Al-Subkī, in the volume he put together on the plague, adds the following:

> Abū Bakr ibn al-ʿArabī's aforementioned view stands. Fakhr al-Dīn al-Rāzī's remarks do not respond to it, because simply noting that each individual in the group that fled is attached to and in love with his worldly life does count as an unusual event that serves as an effective warning, because love for this life is found among those that fled and those that did not. This stands in contrast to understanding the phrase as referring to the great number of people who died all at one time.

It occurred to me that there is another view that avoids the problem laid out by Abū Bakr ibn al-ʿArabī and is different from the view put forward by ʿAbd al-Raḥmān ibn Aslam: The intended meaning of the phrase is that they became united in their judgment to flee. It is possible that some of them did not see fleeing as the best course of action, but only involuntarily left with those who did. Or they expressed hesitation over whether fleeing was the right or wrong choice to make. The phrase would thus convey that they had only eventually united on the view to flee. For this reason, all of them were punished. The Divine warning, that one should not hasten to submit to leaders on an issue like this, would result from consideration of their case. That said, this interpretation does not negate the importance of their numerousness. Furthermore, the phrasing in the verse supports both interpretations, and for one who holds this to be possible, there is nothing to prevent them from interpreting it in both ways.

The fifth is what al-Jaṣṣās notes in the work *The Laws of the Qurʾān*:

> The verse indicates that God, the Exalted, disapproves of their fleeing from the plague, which is equivalent to the following verses: "Say: 'Whether you flee from natural death or from being slain in battle, flight will not profit you'"; and "Wherever you may be, death will overtake you—even

though you be in towers raised high"; and "Say: 'Behold, the death from which you are fleeing is bound to overtake you.'"[20]

4.2

'Umar's Evasion of the Plague in Syria and Other Matters Related to Fleeing the Plague

What follows is a story of 'Umar, who, when he was traveling on the road to Syria, turned around when he heard that the plague had struck there. It also offers a compelling clarification that this was not a case of fleeing from the plague, and that there is nothing in what the reports mention that contradicts that fact.

Sayf recorded:

> The plague occurred in Syria in the months of Muḥarram and Ṣafar, and people died because of it. When it lifted, they wrote 'Umar about it. He set out until he was close to Syria. Then he heard that it was even more severe than before. The Companions of the Prophet advised him that God's Messenger said: "If the plague is in a land, do not enter it. But this command does not apply to you if it occurs in a land you already inhabit." Following this, 'Umar turned back until the plague was lifted there.[21]

Al-Ṭaḥāwī recorded the following account from Anas:

> When 'Umar arrived in Syria, Abū Ṭalḥa and Abū 'Ubayda ibn al-Jarrāḥ met him and told him, "Commander of the Believers! You have the best of the Companions of God's Messenger with you. We just left behind a thing akin to a

burning of fire—that is, the plague. Come back next year." When it was the following year, he came and entered.[22]

Mālik recorded that Ibn 'Abbās said:

'Umar left for Syria. When he reached Sargh, he met the armies' commanders, Abū 'Ubayda ibn al-Jarrāḥ, as well as his colleagues. They informed him that the pestilence had occurred in Syria.

'Umar told me, "Gather the first immigrants who left Mecca to form a new community in Medina together," so I gathered them. He consulted them and informed them that the pestilence had occurred in Syria, and they disagreed about what to do next.

One of them said, "You set out to accomplish a task. We do not see how you can leave it unfinished."

Another said, "You have the rest of the people and the Companions of God's Messenger with you. We do not see how we can proceed into this pestilence."

'Umar replied, "Leave me." Then he told me: "Summon the helpers who aided the first immigrants." I gathered them, and he consulted them, and they acted in the same way as the immigrants and had the same disagreement. He said, "Leave me."

Then 'Umar said, "Summon the leadership of the Quraysh, and those who emigrated after the conquest of Mecca." I summoned them, and not a single one disagreed with the course of action. They said, "We think that you should return with the people and not proceed into this pestilence."

'Umar proclaimed to the people, "I will set out at first light, as shall you!"

Abū 'Ubayda, who was at that time the governor of Syria, asked, "Aren't you fleeing from God's decree?"

'Umar did not like that Abū 'Ubayda had dissented. "Abū 'Ubayda! If only someone else had said this. Yes—we are fleeing from God's decree to God's decree. Let's say you had many camels, and you descended into a valley with two sides, one fertile and the other barren. Is it not the case that if you graze your camels on the fertile side, it is in accordance with God's decree, and if you graze them in the barren side, it is also in accordance with God's decree?"

When ʿAbd al-Raḥmān ibn ʿAwf, who had been absent attending to some need of his, came, he said: "I have some knowledge about this, for I heard God's Messenger saying, 'When you hear that the plague is in a land, do not enter it. But if it occurs in a land while you are there, do not leave it in order to flee from it.'" Then ʿUmar praised God and left.[23]

I would add that al-Dāraquṭnī records this in his *Well-Trodden Paths*:

When ʿUmar intended to turn back at Sargh, he consulted the people. One party, which included Abū ʿUbayda ibn al-Jarrāḥ, said, "Will we flee from death, when we are simply constrained by God's decree? Only what God has written for us will afflict us."

ʿUmar said, "Abū ʿUbayda! If you found yourself in a valley, with one of its two sides fertile, while the other barren, on which of the two will you graze your flock?" He responded, "The fertile side." ʿUmar then said, "We hasten in accordance with God's decree, and if we delayed, it would be with God's decree; we are therefore still within God's decree."[24]

Ibn Khuzayma records this version of the hadith:

When ʿUmar left for Syria and heard about the plague, he groaned. ʿAbd al-Raḥmān ibn ʿAwf told him, "I testify that I heard God's Messenger say, 'When you hear that the plague is in a land, do not enter it. If it occurs when you are in that land, do not leave it in order to flee.'" ʿUmar turned back because of the hadith that ʿAbd al-Raḥmān told him.[25]

HOW 'UMAR'S INDEPENDENT JUDGMENT CONFORMED WITH THE DIVINE WILL

Abū 'Ubayda's consultation with 'Umar on his desire to return goes against the apparent sense of Anas's hadith, mentioned first, in which Abū 'Ubayda and Abū Ṭalḥa advise 'Umar to return. It is possible to reconcile them by supposing that Abū 'Ubayda first gave advice to return, and then realized the value of trusting in God's will when he saw that most immigrants and helpers were inclined to that option, and therefore he retracted his view and shared his change of heart with 'Umar. But when a good argument was made for it, he followed it. Then 'Abd al-Raḥmān came forward with an explicit hadith, and they all changed their minds.

There is another isnad for 'Abd al-Raḥmān ibn 'Awf's report. Mālik recorded it:

> 'Umar ibn al-Khaṭṭāb left for Syria. When he arrived at Sargh, he heard that the pestilence had occurred there. Then 'Abd al-Raḥmān ibn 'Awf told him that God's Messenger said: "When you hear that it is in a certain land, do not approach it. When it occurs in a land while you are in it, do not leave in order to flee from it." 'Umar turned back from Sargh.[26]

Al-Dāraquṭnī records the following version of the ending in his work: "God's Messenger only forbade approaching the land if one hears about the plague. He forbade one to leave it when it occurs in a land while one is in it."[27]

Some people think that this narration conflicts with the first, but this is not the case. Rather, this narration indicates that 'Umar was already inclined to turn around, when he told the people, "I will set out," though without yet having made certain of his decision. Then, when 'Abd al-Raḥmān ibn 'Awf told him the hadith agreeing with his judgment, he praised God for it. Thus, the meaning of the statement, that had 'Abd al-Raḥmān ibn 'Awf not informed him about the Prophet's saying with the hadith, 'Umar would have remained unsure whether to turn around or not. For that reason, he ascribed the cause of his return to ʿAbd al-Raḥmān ibn ʿAwf's hadith, because it is the fundamental precedent on this issue, even if his independent judgment had preceded in conforming to it. For this reason, the incident must be classified as an instance in which ʿUmar's independent judgment conformed with the Divine will.[28]

AL-GHAZĀLĪ'S ACCOUNT OF ʿUMAR'S EVASION OF THE PLAGUE

Al-Ghazālī tells a peculiar version of the story of ʿUmar's evasion of the plague that conflicts with the other accounts we have seen. He writes:

> When ʿUmar and the Companions departed for Syria and reached a place called al-Jābiya, they heard the news that a terrible pestilence and a swift death was there.
>
> The people divided into two groups on what to do. One of them said: "We will not approach the pestilence and cast ourselves to our own destruction."
>
> Another camp said, "On the contrary, we will go, trust in God, and not run away from God's decree nor flee from death. We are like those that God, the Exalted, described: 'Have you not seen those who fled their homes, fearing death, by the thousands? God commanded them, "Die!" but then brought them back to life.'"[29]
>
> They then raised the issue to ʿUmar, and they asked for his view on the matter. He said: "We will return and not go on."
>
> Those that opposed his decision asked him: "Are we not fleeing from God's decree?"
>
> "Yes, we are fleeing from God's decree to God's decree." ʿUmar then offered the following simile to them: "Imagine if there were a flock of sheep that inhabited a valley with two slopes. . . ."

Then al-Ghazālī recounted the rest of the story. He continued:

> Then ʿUmar sought out ʿAbd al-Raḥmān ibn ʿAwf in order to ask him his opinion, but he was missing. When they woke up the next morning, ʿAbd al-Raḥmān ibn ʿAwf came, and ʿUmar asked him his view on the matter.
>
> ʿAbd al-Raḥmān ibn ʿAwf said: "I know something that I heard from God's Messenger."
>
> "Allahu Akbar!" said ʿUmar.
>
> ʿAbd al-Raḥmān went on, "I heard God's messenger saying . . ." and then he recounted the hadith on not entering a land beset by plague.
>
> ʿUmar rejoiced that the hadith agreed with his opinion. The people turned back from al-Jābiya.

This is the context for this story, but, despite my extensive research and investigation, I have not seen anything like it in either the books of hadith or the histories of the conquests. Even if it had been narrated in this form, it is anomalous because parts of it conflict with authentically sourced texts. I only cite it to call attention to the potential benefit it contains. But God knows best.

OTHER VERSIONS OF THE HADITH ON NOT ENTERING A LAND BESET BY PLAGUE

ʿĀmir ibn Saʿd ibn Abī Waqqāṣ said:

> A man came to Saʿd, asking him about the plague, while Usāma ibn Zayd was with him.
>
> Usāma told him, "I will tell you what I heard God's Messenger say: 'This plague is a punishment that was sent against those before you—or upon a faction of the Israelites. It ebbs and flows from time to time. When it occurs in a land while you are in it, do not leave it in order to flee from it. If you hear that it has entered a land, do not go to it.'"[30]

Muslim records a narration from Ibn Jurayj, who cites ʿAmr ibn Dīnār, who said:

> "So do not enter it, and if you enter it, do not leave it in order to flee from it."[31]

Ibn Khuzayma recorded this version that cites Usāma ibn Zayd:

> When the plague was mentioned in the presence of God's Messenger, he said: "If you hear that it is in a land, do not enter it, and if you are already where it is, do not flee from it. It is a punishment that overtook a faction of the Israelites."[32]

Mālik records the following hadith in his work *The Well-Trodden Path*:

> ʿĀmir ibn Saʿd said that he heard his father ask Usāma ibn Zayd: "What have you heard from God's Messenger about the plague?"
>
> Usāma answered: "God's Messenger said: 'The plague was a punishment sent down upon a faction of the Israelites, or those before them. When you hear that it is in a land, do not enter it. If it occurs in a land while you are there, do not leave it in order to flee from it.'"[33]

It seems to be the case—and God knows best—that the reason for the Prophet's statement on the occasion above was that Syria was still, and had been in the times of old, known for having many plagues. When the Prophet entered Tabūk, while raiding Syria, perhaps he heard that the plague was in the direction he had intended and that was the cause of his return without fighting. But God knows best.

Sayf said, in *The Conquests*:

> When Muʿādh ibn Jabal died, ʿAmr ibn ʿAbasa spoke. Then Shuraḥbīl ibn Ḥasana said, "Look at what I say, for God's

> Messenger said: 'If plague strikes in a land while you are in it, do not leave, for death is on your heels. And if the plague is already in a land, do not enter it, for it burns hearts.'"[34]

IF A GREAT DEATH STRIKES, STAY WHERE YOU ARE

Umm Ayman said that she heard God's Messenger give the following advice to some of his family:

> "If a great death strikes a people while you are with them, stay where you are."[35]

The following hadith of 'Ā'isha merits inclusion in this chapter: The Prophet said:

> "Any slave of God who lives in a region in which there is plague who stays put, who does not flee, who acts in patience and in hope of a heavenly reward, will have a heavenly reward like a martyr."[36]

This hadith corroborates one of the two parts of Umm Ayman's hadith: the part that enjoins people to stay put when the plague strikes, which is equivalent to a prohibition on leaving. But God, the Exalted, knows best.

THE PROPHET'S COMPANIONS' DISPUTE ABOUT THE PLAGUE

Sayf ibn 'Umar said, citing his teachers:

> There was a great death during the 'Amwās plague, the likes of which the people had never seen, resulting in emboldening the Muslims' enemies. It persisted for a long time. It got to the point that people started arguing over it

and disagreed among themselves about what to do about it. Muʿādh commanded patience until its purpose became clear. But ʿAmr ibn ʿAbasa commanded retreating from it until its purpose came to light.

Those who wanted to take the path of retreat argued: "People! This is a punishment. It is the great flood that God sent against the Israelites."

Muʿādh and those who viewed patience as the proper course of action responded: "Why do you make your Prophet's prayer and your Lord's mercy a punishment?"

THE CONTEXT OF THE COMPANIONS' DISPUTE OVER THE PLAGUE

Aḥmad said:

ʿAmr ibn al-ʿĀṣ addressed the plague at the end of a sermon he gave to the people: "This is a punishment like fire or flood. The one who steers clear of it, misses it. But it burns and drowns the one who stays."

Shuraḥbīl ibn Ḥasana said: "This is a mercy of your Lord and an answer to your Prophet's prayer, which took the souls of the rightly guided people before you."[37]

Aḥmad recorded a second version:

When the plague struck, ʿAmr ibn al-ʿĀṣ said: "It is such a widespread punishment!"

Shuraḥbīl responded, "I became a Companion of God's Messenger when ʿAmr was more misguided than his family's camel."

Shuraḥbīl added, "It is a mercy of your Lord's, and an answer to a prayer of your Prophet, so unite on its account, and do not divide because of it."

When ʿAmr ibn al-ʿĀṣ heard this, he responded: "He has spoken the truth."[38]

A third version that Aḥmad recorded cited ʿAbd al-Raḥmān ibn Ghanam, who said:

When the plague occurred in Syria, ʿAmr ibn al-ʿĀṣ addressed the people and said the following:

"This plague is a punishment! So disperse into these mountain passes and these valleys."

When Shuraḥbīl heard about this, he got angry. He came out, having torn his robe, carrying his sandal in his hand, and said:

"I became a Companion of God's Messenger when ʿAmr was more misguided than his family's asses. This is a response to your Prophet's prayer, a mercy from your Lord, and the cause of the death of the righteous before you."[39]

Aḥmad records a different hadith on this issue, citing Muʿādh ibn Jabal, who said:

I heard God's Messenger say: "You will emigrate to Syria and conquer it, and there will be among them a disease like buboes or a boil, which pierces people. Through this disease, God will take people there as martyrs and purify their acts."

Ismāʿīl ibn ʿUbaydullāh said: "O God, if you know that Muʿādh ibn Jabal heard it from God's Messenger, then increase in generosity the portion of heavenly reward for him and his family." The plague struck them, and not one of them survived. It pierced his index finger, and he used to say, "By this blood I have the redness of God's grace—nothing delights me more."[40]

Al-Bayhaqī attributes this hadith to Sulaymān ibn Mūsā, who said:

The plague had struck one day at a place called Prostitute's Bridge.*

*Located in southern Syria, near the town of al-Jābiya.

'Amr ibn al-'Āṣ stood and said: "People! This disease is a punishment, so retreat from it."

Shuraḥbīl stood up. "People! I heard one of your Companions say—and by God, I had already converted to Islam and performed the ritual prayer when 'Amr was more misguided than his family's ass—that 'it is a trial that God sent down, so be patient.'"

Mu'ādh stood up next. "People! I have heard the statement of these two Companions of yours. Indeed, the plague is a mercy of your Lord and an answer to the prayer of your Prophet. I have heard God's Messenger saying:

"'You will enter Syria and reside in a place called the Prostitute's Bridge. Ulcerous pustules will emerge among you which will leak puss like the puss of an abscess. God will take you and your offspring as martyrs and purify your actions through it,' Mu'ādh continued, 'Indeed, if only you understood that I heard this from God's Messenger, 'God has given Mu'ādh and his family a generous portion of heavenly reward in the hereafter. . . .'"[41]

Aḥmad recorded a different version from Abū Qilāba, who said:

When the plague struck Syria, 'Amr ibn al-'Āṣ said: "What has occurred is a punishment! So flee from it to the mountain passes and the valleys."

When Mu'ādh heard this, he did not believe it on account of who said it, and responded, "On the contrary, it is a martyrdom, a mercy, and an answer to your Prophet's prayer: 'O God! Give Mu'ādh and his family their portion from your mercy.'"

Abū Qilāba added: "I understood martyrdom and mercy, but I did not understand what the 'answer to the prayer of your Prophet' meant until I was informed that one night when God's Messenger was in prayer, he uttered the following phrase three times in his supplication: 'Give us either the fever or the plague—the fever or the plague!' When he got up in the morning, one of the members of his house said to him, 'God's Messenger! I heard you make a supplication in the night.'

The Prophet asked, 'You heard it?'

'Yes.'

The Prophet said: 'I asked my Lord not to destroy my community in a single year. God granted me that. I then asked Him to not envelop them in sectarianism or allow some of them to harm others. God refused my request. I then asked, 'Then give us either the fever or the plague—the fever or the plague!' three times.' "[42]

Al-Kalābādhī recorded the following hadith that he attributed to Abū Qilāba, who said:

> I heard Abū ʿUbayda and Muʿādh's statement that "this disease is a mercy of your Lord and an answer to your Prophet's prayer." And I used to wonder, "How can this be the Prophet's prayer for his community?" Then one person whom I trust told me this hadith—that he heard that the Prophet said that when Gabriel came to him, Gabriel said:
>
> "Your community's destruction will come about either through the sword or the plague."
>
> Abū Qilāba added: "The Prophet replied by starting to say, 'O God, give us the plague' two times. Then I recognized that this was the prayer that Abū ʿUbayda and Muʿādh spoke about."[43]

Al-Kalābādhī discussed Ibn Isḥāq's narration in the following way:

> The Prophet was informed that the destruction of his community would happen in one of two ways—by the sword or the plague. He knew that one of them, namely, the sword, would either be by way of the religion's disbelieving enemies or through their worldly enemies, such as looting marauders. If either group triumphed over Muslims, they would

> represent the downfall of the religion and the people who safeguard it, as well as the destruction of Muslims' worldly affairs. The Prophet saw that choosing the plague would preserve the religion even if it annihilated some of its people. So he preferred that the community face destruction while safeguarding the religion and its people. . . . It is possible that he only intended by that to obtain martyrdom for his community.

In my opinion, Abū Qilāba does not name his source for the explanation of the Prophet's supplication. The hadith above from Abū Mūsā is more authentic in terms of the content of the hadith and its narrators—that the Prophet prayed:

> "O God, make my community's destruction by the sword *and* the plague!"[44]

We have already seen al-Zamakhsharī's solution—that this is the meaning of Muʿādh referring to "your Prophet's supplication." But there is no contradiction between the two statements, except that, in Abū Qilāba's narration, there is an additional potential cause for the community's destruction. The real difficulty lies specifically in Ibn Isḥāq's narration, because the prima facie sense of it has the Prophet pick only one of the two choices.[45]

The prayer mentioned above has a corroborating hadith from Abū Bakr al-Ṣiddīq, who said:

> I was with the Prophet in the cave, and he said, "O God, give us the sword or the plague!"
>
> I asked, "God's Messenger! I know that you have been asked about the fate of your community. I understand 'the sword,' but what is 'the plague'?"
>
> He replied, "It is cutting like an abscess. If you live long enough, you will see it."[46]

"THE CAUSE OF DEATH OF THE RIGHTEOUS BEFORE YOU"

We have seen explanations of the phrase "a mercy of your Lord and the answer to the prayer of your Prophet," but we have not seen explanations of the phrase "the cause of death of the righteous before you." This is because it does not occur in the narration of Abū Qilāba, recorded by Aḥmad. But it occurs in other narrations that are recorded by different isnads.[47]

Al-Kalābādhī discusses it and said the following:

> It is possible that "the righteous" refers to the Israelites, because they existed before this community, and the plague did strike them.

The hadith occurs in the same context as the story that I cited on the matter involving Balaam.[48] Al-Kalābādhī went on to say:

> The plague was God's purification and expiation of the Israelites because of their silence on what Zimri and others did. The same happened, for instance, when some of them killed others as an act of expiation for those among them who worshipped the calf. When they repented to God and submitted to Him—these are the righteous because they repented, and it is possible that they are the ones referred to in the hadith. But God knows best.

Al-Ṭabarānī records the following involving Muʿādh ibn Jabal, who said:

> God's Messenger said: "You will settle in a place called al-Jābiya. A sickness like the epidemic afflicting camels will strike you there. Through it, God will make you and your descendants martyrs, and purify your actions."[49]

Abū Naṣr al-Tammār said the following involving Mu'ādh:

> When the plague struck Ḥimṣ, one person said that some were saying: "This is the great flood."
>
> When Mu'ādh heard about this, he gave this order: "Gather all of them together in the household of Mu'ādh."
>
> When they had gathered, he said: "This is not the great flood by which Noah's people were punished. Rather, it is martyrdom and a good death."[50]

Ibn Sa'd said:

> When Abū 'Ubayda ibn al-Jarrāḥ was struck with the 'Amwās plague, he appointed Mu'ādh ibn Jabal as the leader.
>
> The disease worsened, and the people told Mu'ādh: "Pray to God to lift this punishment from us."
>
> "It is not a punishment," Mu'ādh said. "Rather, it is the response to your Prophet's prayer, the cause of the death of the righteous before you, and martyrdom meant for those that God has chosen among you. O God, give the family of Mu'ādh their generous share from this Divine mercy."
>
> Mu'ādh was then pierced by the plague.[51]

Al-Bazzār recorded this hadith:

> Al-Ḥārith ibn 'Umayra arrived with Mu'ādh from Yemen. He stayed with him at his house and in his home. The plague struck them, and it pierced Mu'ādh, Abū 'Ubayda ibn al-Jarrāḥ, Shuraḥbīl ibn Ḥasana, and Abū Mālik in a single day.
>
> When 'Amr ibn al-'Āṣ was given news of the plague, he began to raise the alarm among the people: "People! Flee to the mountain trails. There has come down upon you a punishment or plague the likes of which I have never seen."
>
> "You lie!" Shuraḥbīl ibn Ḥasana said to him. "We were the Companions of God's Messenger when you were more misguided than your family's donkeys."
>
> "I speak the truth!" 'Amr said.

Mu'ādh ibn Jabal then said to 'Amr: "No—it's not true. It is neither the plague nor a divine punishment. Rather it is a mercy from your Lord, the answer to the prayers of your Prophet, and the cause of death of the righteous before you. O God, give the family of Mu'ādh a bounteous share from this divine mercy. . . ."

Not a day passed, and the plague struck his son 'Abd al-Raḥmān, the most beloved of all people to him, and the one for whom he was given his patronym. Mu'ādh returned to the mosque and found him there, anxious.

"'Abd al-Raḥmān, how are you?"

"Dear father, 'The truth is from your Lord. Do not be one of the doubters.'"[52]

"As for me," Mu'ādh said, "God willing, you will find me to be one of those who persevere."

'Abd al-Raḥmān died that night and was buried the next day.

Mu'ādh sent al-Ḥārith ibn 'Umayra as a messenger to Abū 'Ubayda to inquire into his well-being. Abū 'Ubayda showed him a lesion on his hand. Al-Ḥārith ibn 'Umayra wept over Abū 'Ubayda, but withdrew from him the instant he saw it. Abū 'Ubayda swore an oath to God that he loved that the redness's blessings had taken a place on his hand.

When al-Ḥārith returned to Mu'ādh, he found him wrapped up. He wept, causing others to weep as well.

Then Mu'ādh regained consciousness. "Dear Ibn 'Umayra! Why did you cry for me? I seek refuge in God from you."

"By God, I did not cry for you."

"Then for whom?"

"I cried because I will no longer be able to glean beneficial knowledge from everything you do."

"Help me sit." Al-Ḥārith helped Mu'ādh sit in his bedroom.

Then Mu'ādh said: "Listen to me, I will give you some parting advice. The one who cries for me because of losing beneficial knowledge from everything I do should realize something: the place of knowledge is only between the two covers of the Qur'an. But, if the meaning of the Qur'an eludes you, seek it from three people after I pass away:

> ʿUwaymir Abū Dardāʾ, Salmān al-Fārisī, and Ibn Umm ʿAbd (he meant ʿAbdullāh ibn Masʿūd). Be wary of the world's traps and the hypocrite's arguments."
>
> Then Muʿādh's death throes intensified. They were the most violent on earth. Every time he regained consciousness from his mortal throes, he would open his eyes and say, "Do You strangle me? I swear by Your might, You surely know that I love You?"[53]

Here is a different version of the hadith, which conflicts with some aspects of the context in the story before it. Aḥmad cited Rāba, who had witnessed the Plague of ʿAmwās and said:

> When the disease flared up, Abū ʿUbayda ibn al-Jarrāḥ stood up and addressed the people with a speech. He declared: "People! Indeed this disease is a mercy from your Lord, the answer to the prayers of your Prophet, and the cause of death of the righteous before you." Then Abū ʿUbayda asked God to reserve for himself a share of heavenly reward in the hereafter for it. Soon after, he was pierced by the plague and died.
>
> Muʿādh ibn Jabal was then appointed as a leader over the people. He stood up to address them after his appointment and said something similar to what Abū ʿUbayda said, but added: "May the family of Muʿādh be given their share of heavenly reward in the hereafter."
>
> Soon after, his son, ʿAbd al-Raḥmān, was pierced by the plague and died. Then he stood up and made a supplication for himself. Then he was pierced by the plague during his sleep. He would say on his death bed: "I do not love anything of this world."
>
> When he died, ʿAmr ibn al-ʿĀṣ stood up to offer a speech, stating: "People! When this disease occurs, it will break out like fire. Seek refuge from it in the mountains."
>
> Abū Wāthila al-Hudhalī said, "By God, I was a Companion to God's Messenger while you were worse than these donkeys here."

> 'Amr answered, "By God, I will not refute what you say, but, by God, we will not stay while it rages."
>
> 'Amr and the people departed and went in different ways. Afterward, the plague lifted. When 'Umar ibn al-Khaṭṭāb heard about 'Amr ibn al-'Āṣ's view, by God, he disapproved of it.[54]

In my view, if this narration is correct, it is possible that 'Amr ibn al-'Āṣ made two addresses: one time when the plague first broke out, in which Shuraḥbīl ibn Ḥasana rebuked him, and another time near the end of it, when Abū Wāthila rebuked him. It is also recorded that 'Umar wrote to Abū 'Ubayda, commanding him to move out with the people to another place. Abū 'Ubayda obeyed him, but was struck before he could move, and the people left after he died. Perhaps 'Amr ibn al-'Āṣ is the one who moved out with them.

Ibn Isḥāq narrated a hadith citing Ṭāriq ibn Shihāb, who said:

> We came to Abū Mūsā while he was in his house in Kūfa so that we could converse in his presence.
>
> When we sat down, he said: "Do not inquire about me, for a man in the house has died because of this poison. It is not blameworthy if you steer clear of this village. So flee to the expanses of your land and its temperate climes, until this trial has lifted. But I will tell you about the attitude the God-fearing detest: the attitude that had one left, the plague would not have struck him. If a devout Muslim does not have this thought, then he is not blameworthy if he leaves and keeps away from it."
>
> Indeed, I was with Abū 'Ubayda in Syria during the year of the Plague of 'Amwās, when the disease broke out. When 'Umar heard about it, he wrote to Abū 'Ubayda, asking him to leave the area. "Peace be upon you," he wrote. "I have a need for you. When you see this letter of mine, do not even put it down until you set out to meet me."
>
> Abū 'Ubayda knew that 'Umar only wanted him to extricate himself from the pestilence. He said: "May God forgive the Commander of the Believers."

Then Abū ʿUbayda wrote to ʿUmar: "Commander of the Believers: I know of your need for me, but I am a part of the Muslim regiment, and I have no desire to leave it, nor will I separate from it until God fulfills His Command and Decree regarding me and them. So release me from your order, Commander of the Believers, and let me and my army be."

When ʿUmar read the letter, he wept.

The people asked him, "Commander of the Believers! Has Abū ʿUbayda died?"

He replied, "No, but it is as if he had."

Then ʿUmar wrote Abū ʿUbayda: "Peace be upon you. You have settled the people in a land that has been spoiled. Take them to a high area that is untouched."

When ʿUmar's letter came to Abū ʿUbayda, he called me and said, "Abū Mūsā! This letter from the Commander of the Believers has come to me, as you can see."

So Abū ʿUbayda went out and scouted a place for the people, so that he could relocate them. I then returned to my residence, and when all of a sudden, I found that my wife had been pierced by the plague, I returned to him and said: "It has struck a member of my family!"

He commanded that a pack animal be made ready to ride. When he put his foot in the stirrup, he was pierced by the plague as well. He said: "By God, I have been struck!" Then he traveled on until he reached al-Jābiya and the pestilence had been lifted from the people.[55]

Al-Bayhaqī records from Qays ibn Muslim, who said, "I heard the following from Ṭāriq ibn Shihāb":

We used to converse with Abū Mūsā al-Ashʿarī. One day, he said to us, "You do not need to inquire about me. This plague has occurred in my own family. If any of you wish to avoid me, he may do so. But beware of two things. First, the one who says, 'The one who flees is thereby safe, while the one who remained behind is thereby afflicted'; and 'if only you had left, you would have been saved, just like that other person was saved when he fled.' Second, the person who says, 'If I had I stayed, I would have been afflicted, just like that other person was afflicted.' I only tell you what is incumbent upon people during the plague."

I was with Abū 'Ubayda when the plague struck Syria. 'Umar had written to him with the following: "When this letter of mine arrives, I order you to come to me. If it comes to you in the morning, do not do anything other than begin riding your mount. If it comes to you in the evening, do not let the night pass without you on your mount making your way to me. There has emerged a situation for which I need you, and only you will suffice regarding it."

When Abū 'Ubayda read the letter, he said, "The Commander of the Believers has sought to delay what cannot be delayed." He wrote him a letter with the following: "I am in the midst of an army composed of Muslims. I do not desire to leave them. I know exactly of the need of the Commander of the Believers, so release me from your order."

When 'Umar received the letter, he wept. He was asked, "Has Abū 'Ubayda died?" He replied, "No, but it is as if he has," meaning that he has drawn close to it.

'Umar wrote him back: "As for Jordan, its land is swamp spoiled by an abundance of humidity. As for al-Jābiya, its land is untouched, so make haste with the Muslims to al-Jābiya."

Abū 'Ubayda then told me: "Set out and settle the Muslims in their new homes."

I said, "I cannot do it."

So he left and started riding out and said to me: "Move the people." Something took hold of him, and he was pierced by the plague. He died as a result, and then the plague was removed.[56]

The following is from al-Haytham's narration:

Abū Mūsā al-Ash'arī said: "Let no one who stayed yet sees the one who left as healthy say, 'If I had left, I would have healed just like so-and-so did.' And let no one who left who was healed and the one who stayed who was stricken say: 'Had I stayed I would have been stricken just like so-and-so.'"

The Muslims hurried to al-Jābiya. Abū 'Ubayda said the following when he read the letter: "We have heard the command of the Commander of the Believers in this, and we obey him. He has commanded me to settle the people on new grounds." Then my wife was pierced by the plague, and I went to Abū 'Ubayda and said, "Someone in my family is exhibiting symptoms of the plague!" He then settled the people in their new homes.[57]

THE MORAL OF THE STORY OF 'UMAR EVADING THE PLAGUE

Abū Mūsā interpreted the prohibition against leaving a country in which the plague occurred as referring to departing a place with the intention of fleeing from the plague, without assigning any intent to that departure other than fleeing it. For example, the prohibition would not apply if the person leaving a town is not one of its residents and therefore found it a disagreeable place to live, so he leaves it for another city that matches the environment of his hometown. What 'Umar wrote in his letter to Abū 'Ubayda ("you have settled a people in a bog") supports this interpretation. The bog's humidity is a sign of its corrupt air, and its rotting stench is because of the abundance of moisture, causing an epidemic of some kind. Thus, the reason that 'Umar gave permission to leave that land was because leaving it was a kind of treatment; he did not give permission to leave purely to flee from death. This is the way his letter to Abū 'Ubayda should be interpreted when 'Umar commanded him to leave the original encampment.

Alternatively, 'Umar understood the prohibition against leaving as principally applying when one's intention in fleeing is purely to evade death. Fleeing for some other reason does not fall under the prohibition. Moreover, his need for Abū 'Ubayda became apparent at the same time, and he hoped, by ordering him to come, he could indirectly keep Abū ʿUbayda safe from that sickness. Abū ʿUbayda immediately understood that this second thing was his primary intent and did not agree with it. ʿUmar then changed his order to include all of those with Abū ʿUbayda; when Abū ʿUbayda objected, he did not see why only he and not his subordinates should be subject to ʿUmar's command.

THE SCHOLARS DIFFER ON THE NATURE OF THE RULING AGAINST FLIGHT FROM PLAGUE

The religious scholars have differed on the prohibition of leaving a town in which the plague strikes. On its face, is it an outright prohibition or something that is just strongly discouraged? There are two views.

Ibn ʿAbd al-Barr said the following:

> The plague is a death that encompasses a land, and therefore it is not permitted for anyone to flee a land in which it occurs if one currently inhabits it. Conversely, one is not permitted to enter the land in permissible which the plague is present if one is outside of it.

Al-Subkī said the following in a volume he gathered together on the plague:

> Our position, which is the position of the majority, is that it is prohibited. . . . Some religious scholars held that it is just strongly discouraged.[58] They agreed on the permissibility of leaving, not in order to flee from death, but to occupy some other land. . . . There is no disagreement on those who leave in order to flee from God's decree of death. There is no way to say that this is something that is not prohibited. Rather, on its face, the debate is regarding those who leave in order to seek treatment.

In my opinion, this framing of the area of disagreement is not apparent. Leaving in order to seek treatment is not forbidden in the view of the Shāfiʿī school and other scholars. Subkī confirmed the view that leaving to avoid God's decree is forbidden. How can he then see the question of whether one leaves in order to seek treatment to be debatable when leaving to seek treatment is not forbidden?

The correct formulation of the issue is to say that the problem is the following: Suppose a person flees a current epidemic with the belief that had God decreed it for him, he would have been struck by it, and with the belief that his fleeing the disease will not save him from God's decree. Nevertheless, he flees, hoping that he will be saved. It is this case that should be disputed. The person who forbids fleeing in the case above cites the aforementioned hadith as proof on this issue. The person who allows it interprets the prohibition as expressing a disapproval but not an outright prohibition, as we discussed earlier.

Ibn Khuzayma, in his *Authentic Hadith*, gave the following as the title for one of his chapters:

> Fleeing from the plague is a mortal sin, and God will punish those who perform this act and will not pardon them.

He used ʿĀʾisha's hadith as proof for this position and indicated that the difference of opinion revolved around the fleeing itself, which is the implication of the reports about ʿUmar and others that we have discussed. But God knows best.

Ibn Abī al-Dunyā recorded a view, attributed to Abū Mūsā al-Ashʿarī, that necessitates the prohibition of fleeing from it:

> That when the plague occurred, al-Mughīra ibn Shuʿba claimed, "Flee from this punishment that has occurred. . . ." I mentioned this to Abū Mūsā, to which he replied: "Abū Bakr said, 'The pious slave said, "O God, the sword or the plague, whatever pleases you most!"'"[59]

The following inference results from bringing this hadith together with the texts above: the Prophet used to prohibit leaving only if it were purely for the purpose of fleeing, and not if it were for seeking treatment.[60]

Abū al-Ḥasan al-Madāʾinī records a case in which a person who fled from plague in order to be safe from it experienced a shortened life. About this, al-Subkī said the following:

> This view has been proven by experience. It is not far from the truth that God made fleeing from it a cause for shortening their lives. The following idea is found in the holy book: that fleeing from jihād is a cause for shortening one's life. God, the Exalted, has said: "Say: 'Fleeing will not benefit you, if you flee from death or fighting, for then you will enjoy but a little.'"[61]

Al-Subkī narrated that his father derived that same meaning from the Qur'anic verse. His father said:

> It is possible that He meant that their survival, even if they lived long after fleeing from death, would bring them little enjoyment in this life in relation to the rewards they would have received in the hereafter.

Ibn ʿAbd al-Barr said the following:

> I have not heard of any scholar fleeing from the plague, other than the one al-Madāʾinī mentioned: "ʿAlī ibn Zayd ibn Jadʿān, who fled Baṣra from the plague to al-Sayāla. He used to attend every Friday prayer in Baṣra and then return to al-Sayāla. When he attended the prayer, they would cry out: 'He fled from the plague!' Then he was pierced by the plague and died in al-Sayāla."[62]

This declaration of lack of sources by Ibn ʿAbd al-Barr is strange because in his *Commentary on Muslim* Qāḍī ʿIyāḍ records that both Masrūq and al-Aswad ibn Hilāl permitted flight from the plague. But it is possible that, even if it can be established that they used to rule that it was permissible to flee the plague, they themselves never fled it.

Al-Madāʾinī recorded the following:

> When the plague had occurred in Cairo, ʿAbd al-ʿAzīz ibn Marwān, who was governor, left it for one of the villages of al-Ṣaʿīd.
>
> One day a messenger from his brother ʿAbd al-Malik came to the village to fetch him. ʿAbd al-ʿAzīz asked him, "What is your name?"
>
> The messenger replied, "Ṭālib ibn Mudrik."
>
> ʿAbd al-ʿAzīz, groaning from illness, said: "I cannot see myself returning to Cairo!"[63]

FLEEING FROM THE PLAGUE IS LIKE FLEEING FROM THE MARCH TO BATTLE

The following addresses this argument: The command against leaving a town in which the plague has occurred—in order to flee from it—amounts to a prohibition. We have already seen the hadiths containing the unqualified command against leaving a place struck by the plague. In some versions, the prohibition is qualified as being limited to leaving with the intent to flee, and the unqualified versions are then interpreted in light of the qualified ones. Regardless, the literal sense of the command is a prohibition.

This construal of the command is strengthened by what Aḥmad records:

> ʿĀʾisha said that God's Messenger said: "The destruction of my community will either be by the sword or the plague."
>
> She continued, "I asked, 'God's Messenger! We know what the sword refers to, but what is the plague?' "
>
> He replied, "A disease that causes buboes of the kind that strikes camels. One who perseveres through it is like a martyr. One who flees from it is like one fleeing from the march to battle."[64]

Al-Bazzār records this hadith in the following form:

> ʿĀʾisha asked, "God's Messenger! We know what the sword refers to, but what is the plague?"
>
> He answered: "It resembles the boils that erupt from the armpits and the groin. It purifies your actions and gives each Muslim an opportunity for martyrdom."[65]

For our purposes here, there is a hadith from Jābir that attests to the versions above. Aḥmad recorded it, citing Jābir ibn ʿAbdullāh that God's Messenger said:

> "Fleeing from the plague is like fleeing from the march to battle. The one who is patient during it is like the one who is patient during the march to battle."[66]

WORDS OF WARNING FOR THOSE FLEEING THE PLAGUE

In *The Conquests*, Sayf records the following, citing ʿAbdullāh ibn Saʿīd, who cites Abū Saʿīd, who said:

> A quick-spreading death struck Baṣra's population. One man from the clan of Tamīm ordered his servant to take his young son, the only child he had, on a donkey, to a prearranged location, until the master caught up with him.
>
> So the servant left with the child in the last part of the night, and his master followed him. Just when the master was about to reach the agreed-upon place, he heard the slave, who had raised his voice: "God does not stop a donkey nor a child from running away with haste! But He greets them in the morning with His decree at the end of a night's revelry."[67]
>
> When the master reached the servant, he asked, "What did you say?"
>
> "I didn't say anything."

But the master knew that the servant wanted him to hear it. He commanded his servant to turn back, and so he did.

Abū al-Tiyāh said:

I asked Muṭarrif ibn ʿAbdullāh ibn al-Shikhkhīr, "What do you think about fleeing from the plague?"

"It is God's decree. You fear it, but there is no fleeing from it."[68]

Al-Jaṣṣās said the following in his book *The Rulings*:

Because the appointed times of death are already determined and defined, there is neither hastening nor delaying what God has decreed. Fleeing from the plague, therefore, is resisting the requirements of the Divine decree, as is acting based on the evil eye, omens, and astrology. All of that is fleeing from what God has decreed and which no one can outrun.

Abū Nuʿaym records the following in *The Ornament*:

Shurayḥ had a brother who had fled from the plague. He wrote him the following letter:

Both you and the place you are currently in are in the
presence of such a Being, that fleeing neither obstructs
Him nor results in escape from Him. Whereas the place
that you left behind neither hastens for a man his fated
death, nor darkens his days. Both you and they are in the
same boat. And yet refuge with One full of power is
always close.[69]

THE SPURIOUS ARGUMENTS OF THOSE WHO PERMIT FLEEING THE PLAGUE

Those who argue that fleeing the plague is permitted first cite a hadith from Abū Hurayra that "the sick should not be received by the healthy."[70] Al-Ṭaḥāwī says the following about this hadith:

> Some scholars hold the view implied by the hadith above and say: "The only reason a plague-ridden place is abhorred is out of fear of contagion." They then ordered the avoidance of and fleeing from places that were diseased. They also offer as evidence 'Umar's returning from Sargh because of the plague . . . and argue: "We have been commanded in these reports not to approach the plague, out of fear for it, specifically the fear that it may infect one who entered the place with it."
>
> But the command to refrain from entering a plague-stricken place—if it were simply based on fear of the plague—would make it permissible for the inhabitants of a place in which it occurred to also leave, because of the rationale it cited. But the inhabitants of a plague-stricken place are forbidden from leaving it. Thus, the reason that they are forbidden from entering it cannot be the reason these scholars give.
>
> In our view, the basis for the prohibition against entering a plague-stricken place—and God knows best—is to prevent the thought "Had I not entered this land, I would not have been struck" should a man enter it and thereby have God's decree for him strike him. Perhaps if he would have remained in the place in which he was, the plague would have also struck him, so he was thereby ordered not to enter, to make the matter of his decreed fate clear.
>
> The same reasoning goes for the command to not leave a plague-stricken place. Doing so would prevent one from thinking: "If I stay in this land, what afflicts its inhabitants will afflict me." Perhaps if he stays, he would not be afflicted at all. Thus, the command to refrain from entering a

place with the plague is for the reason that we have described."

In my view, this argument that al-Ṭaḥāwī describes is illustrated by Abū Mūsā's discussion, which we examined earlier. But the one who thinks it is forbidden to flee generalizes the prohibition as applying to one believing that he escapes death by fleeing and to one who does not believe the matter is settled. The one who thinks it is permissible to flee looks at the reason behind the prohibition and makes it rely on that specific reason. The first approach is more favorable in its enactment of the hadith.

It seems to me that ʿUmar's act of returning before entering the country in which the plague had occurred was not to flee from it at all. His case is the same as a person who intended to enter a house, saw that there was a blazing fire that was impossible to extinguish, and avoided entering it so that it did not strike him. This is a form of precautionary avoidance of dangers that risk life, which is an obligation.

It is clear to me that this was what ʿUmar and those who agreed with him were inclined to do before they heard about the well-authenticated hadith. What they heard confirmed what they had already decided. For this reason, one might say: "ʿUmar returned only because of ʿAbd al-Raḥmān's hadith, not because of what his own analysis of the situation required." The truth, though, is that he already wanted to return, and when he heard the report, it merely strengthened his resolve, as we have already established.

As for those who opposed ʿUmar's view on this issue before they heard the report, they took the path of absolute trust in God, without seeking to examine its reasons. This is a noble station, appropriate for the level of the best Companions. To this end, many of the emigrants to Medina and the helpers took this view, while not a single leader of the Quraysh inclined toward it. ʿUmar only agreed with them because the general welfare of the Muslims dominated his thinking, even though he was one of the most prominent emigrants. The general welfare of Muslims can only be realized by examining reasons and acting in accordance with their most likely outcome, even while believing that all things happen by way of God's decree. This is what is found in the hadith "Tie your camel, but trust in God," which al-Tirmidhī and others record.

To provide context, al-Ṭaḥāwī cites ʿUmar's saying: "O God, the people attribute to me three things, to all of which I plead innocence: they claim that I fled from the plague, to which I plead innocence . . . ," and then he mentions the other two allegations of drinking a type of alcoholic drink and excessive taxation.[71] Al-Ṭaḥāwī continued:

> This is evidence that the reason for his return was for something other than fleeing from the plague. The same thing goes for his letter to Abū ʿUbayda when he ordered him and those of his army who were with him to leave. The reason was only to seek treatment by moving from an unhealthy land to a healthy one.

After providing context of the story of the ʿUraynīs, al-Ṭaḥāwī adds: "Their departure from Medina was to seek treatment and not to flee, which is clear in their story." The same interpretation should be given to what was said concerning ʿUmar's regret for returning from Sargh. Ibn ʿUmar:

> I went to ʿUmar when he arrived in Syria, and I found him talking in his tent. I waited for him in the tent's shadow and heard him crying out while writhing in his sleep: "O God, forgive me for returning from Sargh."[72]

Al-Zarkashī, responding to al-Subkī, said the following in a volume he collected on the plague, quoting from al-Qurṭubī:

> ʿUmar's regret for returning is not authentic. How can he regret doing something that the Prophet commanded? And then retract it and seek forgiveness for it!?[73]

Al-Subkī affirmed al-Qurṭubī's view, but al-Zarkashī rejected it, because he held the hadith's isnad to be authentic. In my view, frankly, I am surprised by al-Qurṭubī. How can well-authenticated reports be rejected in such a way, given the possibility of reconciling the meaning of this hadith with other authenticated reports?

Al-Zarkashī continued:

> It is possible that ʿUmar's regret was out of fear that he was fleeing from God's decree, viewing the command to not enter an area beset by the plague as a dispensation.

Al-Baghawī records the following view:

> The order forbidding flight from the plague amounts to a prohibition, but entering a place beset by plague amounts merely to a reprehensible act that we are ordered not to do, but does not reach the level of being outright prohibited. Meanwhile, entering a place beset by the plague is a license for those who are overcome with trust in God, and turning away from it is a dispensation for the one who chooses to do so.[74]

There is nothing in ʿUmar's discourse that restricts the command to turn away, but it is possible that his regret and seeking of forgiveness is because he went forth on a matter important to the Muslims, arrived at a town for which he had a need, yet returned afterward to Medina because of the hadith he heard that prohibited entering the town. It was possible for him to avoid taking either of these two courses of action: neither not entering the plague-stricken town in compliance with the hadith nor returning to Medina without satisfying the need for which he left Medina. Rather, it was possible for him to take a third course of action: set up camp near Sargh until the plague lifted, and then enter it to accomplish his goal. This is especially the case given that the plague lifted only a short while after his return, as we have seen. The plague lifted after the length of time that it took his letter to Abū ʿUbayda to traverse the road's distance, Abū ʿUbayda's response, then his second letter to him commanding him to change the army's placement, then the latter's compliance with his command, and his commencing to transfer the army.

Perhaps he thought it would have been better had he waited for the plague to lift before his return, because his return with the army that accompanied him would have been a hardship on him and on them. No report exists recording a command to return; rather, there is a command against entering or approaching a place beset by plague. This is according to the phrasing of the report itself, insofar as it contains the phrase "do not enter" or "do not approach." Therefore, it is possible that his regret was for this reason.

Qāḍī ʿIyāḍ notes the following when he mentions the dispute among the emigrants to Medina and those who helped them on the issue of returning:

> The argument for both groups is clear, because it is built on fundamental principles of the Shariʿa. The first is trusting God and accepting his decree and design; the second is exercising restraint and precaution in avoiding recklessly exposing oneself to life-threatening situations.

Both of these are subsidiary principles derived from the fundamental principle of Divine decree. It is sometimes said: "ʿUmar's return was only because of the hadith." This is because he would not have returned based on mere opinion without a valid religious proof. We have just discussed this above.

Certainly, there exist explicit reports on individuals other than ʿUmar acting based on only trusting in God. Ibn Khuzayma records this hadith:

> Al-Zubayr ibn al-ʿAwwām went out raiding near Egypt. The authorities in Egypt wrote to him saying that the plague had occurred in the land and not to enter it. Al-Zubayr replied: "I have gone out to war on account of the sword and the plague." So he entered Egypt, and was pierced on the brow between his eyes, yet recovered.[75]

The word "recovered" means that he recovered from his illness.[76] Abū Mijlaz, a well-known Successor, said:

> When the plague occurred and disappeared from Baṣra, they counted those who recovered from it, and the total was a certain number.

Abū Mūsā added, "The specific word for 'recovered' means that they were healed completely of the plague. . . . It is said that this term is used for those who recover from a sickness that usually strikes a person once in their life, such as smallpox." But God knows best.

I would add that Ibn Abī al-Dunyā recorded a report, in his work *The Book of Illness and Expiations*, that Abū Mijlaz used to say:

> "When conversing with the sick, say only what will please the one who is ill."
>
> He would come to me when I was pierced by the plague and say: "They counted so and so in the neighborhood as recovered, and they counted you as among them . . . and I would rejoice at that."[77]

A NOTE ON CONTAGION

Al-Bayhaqī recorded another report involving al-Zubayr that conflicts with this one. Al-Zubayr's son, ʿUrwa, said:

> When I was a boy, one day I met my father, al-Zubayr, who had a leper beside him. I wanted to touch the leper, but al-Zubayr pointed at me and ordered me back, out of disgust with me touching him.[78]

In my view, there is no contradiction between this hadith and the one we discussed earlier. Rather, al-Zubayr's choice to approach the man with leprosy was based on the strength of his faith and the sureness of his certainty. He forbade his young son from touching the man with leprosy out of fear that God would decree that it afflict him, and al-Zubayr thought that his son's ignorance would lead him to think that the cause of the affliction was the touching, and he might believe in the type of causal transference in which it is forbidden to believe. We will address this topic in detail under the third issue.

A second issue that al-Subkī reports is that those who permitted fleeing from the plague used to cite as evidence the analogy of fleeing from lions or fleeing from an enemy whom one is not able to fend off. It is permissible, for instance, those fundamentally incapable of resisting infidel armies and brigands to retreat. On this, he quotes Abū al-Ḥasan al-Kiyā al-Harrāsī, who claims a consensus of the Shāfiʿīs, saying:

> We do not know of any view opposing the permissibility of withdrawing, even though it is the case that one's life span neither increases nor diminishes due to human action.

The answer to this spurious argument, according to al-Subkī, is the following:

> The analogy for the permissibility of fleeing from the plague based on fleeing from lions and enemies is weak, because safety from the latter is rare and dying from these is assured, such that the case becomes like the one who casts himself into fire. These cases are unlike fleeing from a town in which the plague occurs, because safety from it is very possible, even if it is not probable.

My assessment of the analogical argument is that it has an element that distinguishes it from fleeing the plague. The issue of standing still in front of a lion as it attacks falls under the prohibition against exposing oneself to destruction. Meanwhile, the command against fleeing from the plague is clear. So how can the two be equal?

The third issue involves drawing an analogy to justify the absolute permissibility of leaving a plague-ridden place to the story of the ʿUraynīs who left land with an unhealthy climate. The response is as follows: The act of leaving is a type of seeking of medical treatment, or a sick person refraining from foods that do not agree with him, because there is no difference between foods and airs in their effect on the sick. Therefore, the act of leaving a land that does not agree with the constitution of the sick is a type of seeking of medical treatment, which it is permissible to do.

Al-Subkī said the following:

> I think that there is a problem with this response. In my opinion, this is because its form allows one to respond, "The plague also originates in corrupted air. Therefore, it must be the case that leaving the town in which it is found is absolutely permissible, just as it was permissible for the ʿUraynīs."

And this is not in accordance with the truth of what we have discussed earlier—that the plague stems from the pricks of the jinn. The truth is that the ʿUraynīs leaving was not ever for the purposes of fleeing, but only to seek treatment, as we saw from what al-Ṭaḥāwī recorded. Their leaving was because of an existing necessity. Their camels were not used to living in the town. The illness came from their grazing, and the effects of their illnesses were in their urination, their milk, and their breathing in of the air. Therefore, leaving this area is implicit in the command to support one's existence. This stands in contrast to leaving an area in which the plague had occurred for another area where it had not. This departure is motivated by speculation, because one cannot be certain that the plague will not occur in the other area as well.

There is something else that strengthens the distinction between fleeing from the plague and leaving an unhealthy place. The totality of the principles of medicine boil down to one's natural and customary habits. The ʿUraynīs were Bedouin and countryfolk, as it is explicitly mentioned in some versions of reports about them. Their natures did not agree with urban living. Thus the Law-Giver advised them to seek treatment with what restored them in terms of their nature as Bedouins.

It is from this perspective that one may understand 'Umar's command to Abū 'Ubayda to move his army from the place they had first decamped to another place better suited to their natural constitutions. Farwa ibn Musayk's hadith is pertinent to this point:

> I asked, "God's Messenger! We have a place that is named Abyana, which is the land of our countryside and our sustenance, but it is pestilential."
>
> The Prophet replied: "Leave it. For destruction lies in what causes sickness."[79]

Ibn Qutayba notes that "what causes sickness" indicates its proximity to pestilence. Al-Khaṭṭābī says that this hadith does not address contagion, but rather the matter of treatment. The rectification of the airs is one of the most commonplace things when it comes to physical wellness. The corruption of the airs presents one of the most harmful risks to good health and is that which the doctors consider the most efficient causes of sickness. Of course, all of that is through the permission and will of God, the Exalted, glory be to Him.

The fourth issue is what al-Zarkashī notes: Those who permit fleeing the plague without qualification cite as an analogy the permissibility of fleeing from the leper. He means by this the hadith that al-Bukharī recorded from Abū Hurayra, who said:

> God's Messenger said: "There is no such thing as contagion, nor is there evil augured from a croaking crow, a death-bird, or a stomach-serpent. But flee from the leper just as you flee from lions."[80]

It is also recorded in Muslim's *Authentic Hadith*:

> There was a leper in Thaqīf's delegation, and the Prophet sent the following message through a messenger: "We have made the oath of loyalty with you, so return."[81]

Abū Dāwūd also records a hadith citing Ibn ʿAbbās:

> The Prophet said: "Do not stare at lepers."[82]

There are two ways to respond to this. The first is Ibn al-Ṣalāḥ's approach. Following others, he reconciled the contradiction with the apparent meaning of Abū Hurayra's hadiths—two of which say, "Do not bring the sick to the healthy" and "Flee from the leper the same way you flee from a lion"—with the other hadith that says, "There is no contagion." He argued:

> One way to reconcile their apparent contradiction: These diseases are not contagious per se, but God makes the intermixing of the sick with the healthy a cause for the transmission of illness. In some cases, it fails to occur as an effect of its cause, just as is the case in all causes.
>
> As for the hadith that claims, "There is no contagion," it is a negation of what the pre-Islamic people believed—that the contagion happens naturally. It is for this reason that the Prophet, in response to those who said that contagion exists, asked, "Then, who infected the first?"
>
> Here is another way to reconcile this apparent contradiction: Know that God makes mixing with the sick the cause of sickness, and He gave warning about the harm, which, most of the time, is the consequence of an illness' presence, by way of God's act, may He be exalted.

Our teachers confirmed this in their later summaries of this material. But one of them, al-Bulqīnī, said the following:

> A better way of expressing it would have been to change "God makes mixing with the sick the cause of sickness" to "sometimes God makes mixing with the sick the cause of sickness."

This is a valuable clarification, because it can be imagined that this occurs always or predominantly, but the reality deviates from this.

The fundamental principle concerning this matter is expressed by al-Shāfiʿī's opinion:

> The medical experts and observers claim that lepers oftentimes will infect their spouses. Moreover, this is an illness that prevents coitus. No man's soul comes close to desiring copulation with one afflicted with it. Nor does a woman's soul desire to have sex with one who has it. As for the offspring, it is clear—and God knows best—that when it is born, it contracts leprosy. Few children are safe from it, and for those who are saved, it still reaches their progeny. We ask God, by His Bounty and Generosity, for a cure for it.[83]

Al-Bayhaqī added the following to al-Shāfiʿī's opinion:

> But it has been established from the Prophet that he said, "There is no contagion." However, the Prophet meant to counteract what people used to specifically believe, in the age of ignorance before Islam, that an act can be attributed to things other than God, the Exalted; and that sometimes He makes, through His will, the intermixing of the healthy with the sick a cause for the origination of that sickness. For this reason, the Prophet said: "Do not bring the sick to the healthy." He also said the following about the plague: "Whoever heard about it in a certain land should not enter it." Other hadiths have a similar meaning. But all of that is through God's decree, may He be exalted.

What is apparent to me is that al-Shāfiʿī did not narrate the hadith negating contagion, the explanation of which I will discuss shortly. For this reason, he depended on the claims of the doctors and the medical observers and others who did not address the interpretation of the hadith.[84]

Al-Bukhārī and Muslim recorded a version of this hadith:

> A man from the Bedouin came to the Prophet and said, "The first bit of mange starts at the camel's lip, then it affects all the camels."

God's Messenger asked, "Then who infected the first?"[85]

According to Ibn Masʿūd:

> God's Messenger said: "One thing does not transmit diseases to another."
>
> To which a man from the Bedouin replied. "God's Messenger! The first bit of mange starts at the camel's lip or his tail, and soon it is a catastrophe for the camels, all of whom become mangy."
>
> God's Messenger answered: "There is no such thing as contagion, nor a death-bird, nor a stomach-serpent. God created each soul, and foreordained their life spans, their livelihoods, and their hardships."

Ibn Khuzayma cited this hadith and followed it with this section heading: "On the report narrated from the Prophet in which he commands fleeing from lepers: I fear that some people may take this to affirm that diseases are contagious, but I do not think this is the case, may God be praised." Then he recorded this hadith from ʿĀʾisha, who said:

> God's Messenger said: "There is no contagion. But when you see the leper, flee from him just as you would flee from lions."[86]

But there is also Jābir's hadith, in which "the Prophet took a leper's hand and placed it along with his own in a large bowl, then said, 'In the name of God, depending on Him, and having trust in Him.'" In another version:

> We were with the Prophet, who was eating, when a leper came. He said: "Come near and eat," while relying on God and putting trust in Him.

Ibn Khuzayma explained it in the following way:

> Out of his mercy and kindness for his community, the Prophet ordered them to flee from the leper, just as, out of

> sympathy for them, he prohibited introducing a sick animal to the healthy. He also ordered them to flee from the leper out of fear that some Muslims would suppose that one who approaches a leper gets leprosy or that healthy livestock become ill after mixing with sick livestock. He also did so out of fear that some Muslims would suppose that the person afflicted with leprosy was infected by a previous person, just as they wrongly infer that, in the case of livestock, when mange affects them, the sick among the livestock were the first to transmit it to them. In these ways, the idea of contagion, which the Prophet denied, could take root.
>
> After negating these notions, the Prophet said: "No one thing transmits disease to another." He commanded them to avoid that notion so that Muslims may find refuge in the truth from the falsehood of affirming contagion. The Prophet taught that an evil omen is something they find in their hearts, then he taught that trusting in God consists in leaving such omens behind.
>
> This is likewise the case with lepers and leprosy. The one who is weak in trusting in God, if he is struck with leprosy after having gotten close to a leper, will then believe in contagion and evil omens, because of the weakness of his trust in God and because the Prophet supposedly affirmed contagion when he commanded one to flee from the leper and because he sent the leper away. What further supports the reconciliation of this apparent contradiction as well as the negation of contagion is the fact that the Prophet ate with the leper by having faith and trust in God. . . .
>
> As for the command against staring at the leper, it is consistent with the above. It is possible that its meaning is that the leper will feel depressed and dislike that healthy people stare at him, because there are few experts who have a treatment for it, other than covering it up. Even if this were not the case, the leper would still prefer to cover up his affliction.

This is the most accurate and fitting interpretation. It is better than the synthesis of the conflicting hadiths that al-Bayhaqī noted. Ibn al-Ṣalāḥ and those after him adopted this approach, because, at its root, it negates contagion, just as the authentic reports clearly state. The reports that present the opposite, which the latter are combined with—those which largely affirm contagion—were interpreted in accordance with the intent to settle the issue.

Mālik noted, when he was asked about the hadith on staring at lepers:

> I have not heard that others see it as a basis for disapproval, I see the texts with the command to not stare as expressing fear that an objectionable belief would arise in the believer's heart.

Mālik means that belief in contagion would arise in him. As for the hadith that al-Bayhaqī recorded:

> God's Messenger said: "There is no contagion. It is not permissible to take the sick to the healthy, but it is permissible for the healthy to do as he pleases."
>
> He was asked, "Why is that so, God's Messenger?"
>
> The Prophet said: "It is harmful."

This hadith is weak.[87] But assuming that the text of the hadith is well-preserved, the pronoun in the text "it is harmful" refers to the sickness, and undoubtedly, sicknesses are harmful. The pronoun cannot refer to the act of taking the healthy to the sick. If that were so, it would entail affirming contagion, which is negated in the beginning of the hadith. The issue thus circles back to the earlier interpretation. But God knows best.

In his work *The Meaning of Reports*, al-Ṭaḥāwī adopted the method taken by Ibn Khuzayma in reconciling the apparent contradiction. He cites the hadith that states "Do not take the sick to the healthy," then notes the following:

> Its meaning is that when a healthy person is afflicted with that disease, the one who took them may say: "If I had not taken the healthy to the sick, then the healthy would not have been afflicted with this illness." But the reality is that, even if he had not taken the healthy to the sick, the illness

would have afflicted him because of God's decree of it. So the Prophet forbade taking the healthy to the sick so that this mistaken idea, from which most people are not immune, would not occur in their hearts. . . .[88]

The Prophet negated contagion and retorted, "Who transmitted the disease to the first?" By this, he meant that if the second is afflicted only because of transmission from the first, what thing transmitted that to the first? There was nothing to transmit it to him. But, if what afflicts the first is through God's decree, this likewise is what afflicts the second. . . . It is possible to interpret the Prophet's saying, "There is no contagion" as a negation of serial transmission without a beginning. And it is also possible to interpret his saying, "Do not take the sick to the healthy" as motivated by the Prophet's fear that, if one takes the healthy to the sick and, by God's decree, the same illness that afflicted the first then afflicts him, then the idea would occur to him that the first one's illness was transmitted to him. Thus, the Prophet disliked taking the sick to the healthy, out of that fear. But God knows best.

Al-Jaṣṣāṣ followed al-Ṭaḥāwī in this regard:

Meanwhile, al-Bayhaqī brought into harmony two other hadiths. The first, in which he sent "a leper in Thaqīf's custody" away, and the second, in which he put the leper's "hand in the bowl." He brought these together by saying that the latter is addressed to a person who is able to patiently bear hardships and surrender choice in matters of God's decree. The former is addressed to one who fears that he is unable to patiently bear hardships, so he is cautious of the types of things that God's law allows one to be cautious about.[89]

Al-Qurṭubī responded to this difficulty in his work *The Discerning*:

The prohibition is only against taking the sick to the healthy for fear that the belief that occurred to people in the age of

> ignorance before Islam might occur, or for fear of the self's capacity for delusions and imagination's influence. This is similar to the Prophet's saying, "Flee from the leper," because even if we believe that leprosy does not transmit to others, we find an aversion and abhorrence of it in ourselves, such that a person himself is disgusted by approaching or sitting with the leper; that person thinks to himself that perhaps he will suffer because of it. This being the case, it is clear that it would be better for a person not to expose human beings to that which requires a spiritual struggle. Rather, he should avoid the paths that cause false supposition and distance himself from the causes of pain, even while knowing that fear does not save one from an occurrence of Divine decree. But God knows best.

Then I found the one who preceded everyone else on this issue, Abū ʿUbayd al-Qāsim ibn Salām, who noted that the meaning of the prohibition of taking the sick to the healthy is not to affirm contagion. Rather, it is because if the healthy got sick through God's decree, the idea that it was because of contagion may occur to the one who got sick. He is thereby put to a spiritual test and begins having doubts in his belief in God's decree. For this reason, the Prophet commanded one to avoid the practice. In Abū ʿUbayd's own words:

> A certain person interpreted the hadith as motivated by fear for the healthy on the part of those that have the sickness. . . . This is a wicked interpretation of the hadith because it is a license to engage in illicit omens. The proper understanding of the Prophet's prohibition of taking the sick to the healthy is, in my view, what I just discussed—to avoid having doubt in God's decree.

4.3
The Wisdom of Prohibiting Flight from a City Afflicted by Plague

Some scholars held the view that the prohibition is a religious one, with no intelligible reason behind it. Even though there is an obligation to flee from all kinds of life-threatening dangers, they reasoned that the prohibition against leaving a city that has been afflicted by the plague is still valid. Therefore, there must be a hidden reason for the prohibition, which cannot be known. Thus, in this case, it is more appropriate to simply accept and comply with what the Divine Law-Giver has commanded.

Many, however, held the view that the prohibition is susceptible to rational analysis, and they highlight the wisdom behind it. For example, in most cases, the plague is widespread in the place where it strikes, such that when it strikes and an individual is afflicted by it, then it is quite clear that death's rope has ensnared him, and his fleeing will not benefit him. Indeed, if his time has come, he will die, regardless of whether he stays behind or flees, or vice versa.

Those who favor this latter position proceed to note that the legal acts of the healthy in a city afflicted by the plague are of the same status as the acts of those who are terminally ill, a topic we will discuss in detail in the fifth chapter. When the sickness has taken hold of a certain person, there is no escaping from it, and remaining is the right course of action because leaving is futile; an act not worthy of reasonable people.

Furthermore, if people flee in successive waves, they will leave behind those afflicted with plague who are too weak to leave. The welfare of the sick will be ruined because there will be no one to take care of them; the fate of the dead is similar, since there will be no one to prepare them for burial. The leaving of the strong on a journey breaks the heart of one who does not have the strength to do so. As it is said concerning the wisdom of the threat of severe punishment for those fleeing from the battlefield: fleeing fills those who remain in the battle with fear, alarm, and defeat.

Al-Ghazālī has harmonized the two seemingly contradictory positions in his work *The Revival.* He holds:

> The corrupt air does not harm insofar as it comes into contact with the exposed part of the body, but rather insofar as it is repeatedly inhaled and thereby reaches the lungs and the heart and affects them. Only after affecting the inside of the body does the illness show its effects on the outside. The one who leaves the city that is afflicted by the plague, in most cases, has not been rescued from the thing that has taken root from before, but has only deluded himself about his safety and, in his delusion, compromised his reliance on God. . . . If the healthy were allowed to leave, then no one would be left to attend to the sick, and their welfare would be ruined.

Another aspect of the wisdom behind this prohibition—which we discussed earlier—is that the one who leaves might say, "If I had not left, I would have died," and the one who remains might say, "If only I had left like that person, I would have been safe." To say "if only I had . . ." encourages a kind of thinking that is condemned. Ibn ʿAbdAbd al-Barr was inclined to this opinion:

> The prohibition against leaving a place beset by plague is based on faith in God's decree. The prohibition against entering is to avoid blaming oneself.

Ibn ʿAbd al-Barr also quotes Ibn Masʿūd:

> The plague is a trial for the one who stays and the one who leaves.

Ibn ʿAbd al-Barr also mentioned something similar to what we have seen, but added:

> Leaving a place beset by plague is fleeing from the judgment that God has decreed and that He commanded one to endure patiently, and for whom He made the heavenly reward for any resulting death akin to the reward of the martyr.

The one who stays patiently, resigned to God's will, gets the reward of a martyr even if he does not die by the plague, as we have discussed earlier. But in fleeing from something like that, there is a large loss in heavenly reward, along with ignorance of whether he is truly safe from the death that he is fleeing, as God, the Exalted, has said, "Say: Fleeing, if you flee from death or fighting, will not benefit you, for you only tarry but for a little."[90]

Ibn al-ʿArabī said:

> The wisdom of the prohibition from fleeing is that if he does not die when he flees, he attributes it to his escape from the plague, when, in fact, it was but a moment he lived through. Everything that is found as contemporaneous to causes should not be attributed to them, but only to that which the Divine law attributes to them. It is said: "Fleeing is forbidden for him because the cause of the disease has already ensnared him through God's judgment." And it is said: "Fleeing is forbidden so the sick would not be left without a caretaker. . . ." As for the wisdom of preventing someone from entering a place beset by plague, I think that God commanded it so that no one exposes himself to death, even if there is no security from God's decree except through the type of vigilance that God allows.
>
> Another form of wisdom in God's command to deny entering a place beset by plague is protecting someone from committing the sin of ascribing partners to God. It makes it so one may not say: "If only I had not entered that place beset by plague, I would not have gotten sick" or "If only so-and-so had not entered that place, he would not have died. . . ." It is said: the wisdom in the prohibition against entering a place beset by plague is so that the false ideas which cling to those that enter would not be more than false ideas which cling to the one who leaves. But God knows Best.[91]

Then I found an excellent chapter on this topic by Ibn Daqīq al-ʿĪd:

> My view, concerning the reconciliation of the prohibition against fleeing from a country that is afflicted by the plague with the prohibition from entering that same place is that, in entering it, one exposes oneself to an affliction that is perhaps unbearable—perhaps the kind that calls upon someone to practice a high level of patience and trust in God. Such a person may refuse to acknowledge this reality out of the self's delusions and motivations, which he has not considered carefully enough to know the truth. But God knows best.
>
> As for the wisdom of the prohibition against fleeing a place beset by plague: In some cases, one may understand it as undue preoccupation with causes. Consider the case of one who tries to secure safety as best he can: He encounters difficulty in entering just as he encounters it when fleeing. He is therefore commanded to refrain from the difficulties in both courses of action. The Companion had alluded to what we just mentioned in the hadith concerning the two sides of the valley, one fertile, one barren, when he asked: "Shall we flee from God's decree?"
>
> The Prophet's saying confirms this point. He said: "Do not desire to meet the enemy, but when you do meet them, be patient." He commanded them to abstain from desire to meet the enemy, out of fear of exposing themselves to a kind of tribulation and self-delusion, as no one is safe from the self's trickery when it occurs. Then he ordered them to be patient when they did meet the enemy, fully accepting of God's command, may He be exalted.[92]

I have also seen what Ibn Abī Jamra has said on this matter, which I summarize here:

> The Prophet's saying "Do not hasten to a place beset by plague" is a prohibition of opposing the Divine decree, and it contains much wisdom. The same theme is present in

> God's statement: "Do not, by your own hands, cast yourselves to perdition."[93]
>
> Jesus, upon him be peace, has said: "The master tries the slave, and it is not for the slave to try the master." Add to this the statement: "Do not leave, fleeing from it." In this, there is guidance that one should suffer what has been decreed and be content with it. In addition, when a trial descends, it targets the people of a locale, not the locale itself. Whoever God wishes to strike with a trial or tribulation, he will be struck without a doubt; no matter where one turns, it will find him. Thus, the Law-Giver guides one to wish for nothing other than to refrain from exhausting oneself by fleeing, and God knows best.
>
> And among other reasons not to flee are what one of the physicians has asserted: that in the country in which a pestilence occurs, the humors of the people adapt to the air of those places and absorb it into their own temperaments, and thereby it becomes like what is healthy air for others. But if they move to places with healthy air, it does not suit them. Rather, when they breath in the healthy air, it ushers to the heart the malicious vapors to which the body had adapted. When it reaches the heart, the very illness that they were fleeing from strikes them. So the Prophet prohibited their flight on these grounds.

This opinion from a physician, in addition to what we already discussed, is, first of all, built on the facts that both the plague and the pestilence are the same in this regard, and that the cause of the plague is the air's corruption rather than the pricks of the jinn. But we have given an opposing account of this in the last part of the first chapter. The most reliable view concerning the wisdom of preventing entrance while prohibiting fleeing from places beset by plague is what was relayed from Ibn Khuzayma, al-Ṭaḥāwī, and Ibn ʿAbd al-Barr. But God, Glorified and Exalted, knows best what is correct.

CHAPTER FIVE

WHEN THE PLAGUE STRIKES

5.1
What Responses to the Plague Are Lawful?

In the previous chapters, we saw the command to refrain from leaving a town stricken by plague in order to flee it, and the injunction to stay in the town in patience and hopeful of heavenly reward, knowing that one will not be afflicted by anything other than what God has decreed. Now we will discuss a number of issues that are related to when a plague occurs in a town, generally. After that, I will discuss the problems that are related to when the plague afflicts the individual.

It is immediately incumbent on anyone who has been hurt by the plague to rectify wrongs that they have committed against others, discharge any remaining duties, repent from transgressions against God, express regret for past sins, and not to lapse into injustice or deviance. This is demanded at all times, but it is especially emphasized when a plague occurs and has become widespread, and for any individual who is specifically afflicted with it.

PRAYING TO GOD TO LIFT THE PLAGUE

Question: Is praying to God for plagues to be lifted countenanced in the law? If it is, does the law countenance that such prayers be conducted in groups, or should everyone pray individually in accordance with what suits them? If the law authorizes group prayer, must it be performed in the manner specific to the qunūt,*

---

*Qunūt is a special supplication that may be performed as part of the formal prayer ritual (ṣalāt). Depending on one's school, it is performed either immediately before or after the bending down motion of the prayer (rukūʿ), while the one praying is in a standing position.

as is the case with other calamities, as some authorities hold, or does the law demand that the gathering take place outside of the town in the surrounding desert after fasting, as is the practice when performing the prayer for rain in a time of drought?

Answer: Praying to God by performing the qunūt prayer for the plague to be lifted from Muslim lands where it has spread is authorized by the law, especially for followers of the Shāfiʿī school. This holds whether it is performed as a group or by individuals on their own, based on the view that the plague is a type of calamity. Al-Shāfiʿī was of the view that performing the qunūt prayer is authorized whenever a calamity occurs, and al-Rāfiʿī and others specifically mentioned pestilence and famine as examples of calamities. One group of Shāfiʿīs holds that the plague is a type of pestilence, as we saw in the first chapter. Thus, it follows that performing the qunūt prayer to ask for deliverance from the plague is authorized in the law.

Al-Shāfiʿī said in *The Source*:

> I have no objection to performing the qunūt prayer when a calamity occurs, but I do object if it is performed in the absence of a calamity.

However, a later follower of the Shāfiʿī school equivocated on this issue and gave no answer. He reasoned that the plague is more specific than the pestilence and occurred during the time of the righteous Companions, then again in the time of the righteous generation that followed the Companions. Yet there are no reports of any of them performing the qunūt to ask for deliverance from the plague.

This position that the later follower of the Shāfiʿī school holds is problematic because its reasoning requires impeaching the validity of performing the qunūt for calamities, not just in the particular case of the plague. The permissibility of performing the qunūt upon the occurrence of a calamity is a position that Shāfiʿī, may God be pleased with him, the founder of the school, expressly held, which binds those who follow him to profess this view. It may be the case, however, that this later follower adopted that opinion of his own accord, not on the school's authority, in which case this later follower's argument is internally consistent.

The very same argument that he offered in support of the qunūt prayer's invalidity for plagues was made by the Ḥanbalī author of *The Positive Laws* to show that the performance of the qunūt prayer for calamities is not authorized. He said:

> The clearest position is that the qunūt should not be done for deliverance from pestilence because there are no reliable reports that the qunūt was performed for the ʿAmwās plague, nor for any other plague.

Indeed, only the Shāfiʿīs deem the qunūt to be authorized for calamities. As for supplicating in general, the best-supported view is that it is authorized. In fact, it is preferred that those in territories free from pestilence pray for those in territories that suffer from it, just as it is preferred that those in fertile lands pray for those in drought-stricken lands.

One of the Ḥanbalīs disputed this. I read in a volume put together by al-Manbijī that praying for the plague's lifting is not approved of, because Muʿādh refused to do it on account of the fact that death from plague offered a martyrdom, a mercy, and a fulfilment of our Prophet's prayer for his community. Al-Manbijī added:

> If the qunūt prayer were authorized, Muʿādh would not have required them to ask him. Furthermore, he would have done it himself of his own accord. Were the qunūt authorized, he would have immediately done it when the people asked him to do it based on what they thought was in their best interests. Were it not for the fact that the qunūt was not authorized, he would have hastened to acquiesce to their request. Citing the precedent of the validity of prayer asking God to lift the fever is no rebuttal to this view, because dying from a fever is rare, in contrast to the plague, which is usually lethal. Thus, praying for deliverance from the

> plague would essentially be seeking deliverance from death. But death is a decreed inevitability whose occurrence can neither be quickened nor delayed even for a blink of an eye.

Al-Manbijī's argument is weak. Citing God's decree as a reason to abandon supplication would require abandoning supplication in all matters and, in fact, leaving off purposeful action altogether. Qāḍī ʿIyāḍ ascribed this view to a Sufi and rejected it out of hand. Furthermore, the hadiths establishing the authorization of praying to God to give health and healing to the sick, to seek protection from madness, leprosy, and other harmful illnesses, and to seek protection from bad character traits, evil actions, lower desires and diseases that are too many to enumerate and too well-known to mention.

Likewise, clinging to God's decree in this sense would require abandoning treatment for sicknesses even though authentic hadiths authorize and permit it, and even though there is no doubt that seeking treatment through prayer is more effective than seeking treatment through natural substances. Moreover, the plague is not death, it is but one sickness among others. One should pray for the plague to be lifted and seek protection from it, as is the case with all sicknesses, even if plague expiates sins and some die a martyr's death from it. As we have already seen, it is caused by the pricks of the jinn, and we are commanded to seek protection from them.

Finally, no believer may pray for another to be afflicted by the plague because it is calling for an affliction that would be widespread. Doing so is prohibited, even if it contains the possibility of martyrdom, as is the case with a flood or a widespread disaster or other similar things; it is not permissible to pray for them to occur to others. In fact, there is more widespread harm in the plague than in a flood. Likewise, no Muslim may pray for others to get sick, even if the one afflicted may obtain much heavenly reward in abundance.

As a subsidiary issue, it is not permissible for any Muslim to pray for another's death without a qualifying reason. In al-Karābīsī's discussion in *The Etiquette of Judges*, one senses that he thinks such a practice is disapproved of, but not quite prohibited. He said: "If one person prays for the death of another, he is not to be given a discretionary punishment." It is possible that al-Karābīsī thought that the time of death cannot be hastened nor delayed and did not think the prayer had any effect in hastening it.

Al-Millawī compiled a volume on prayers for lifting pestilence, which he named *The Seed of Excellence in Deliverance from the Pestilence.* He delimited the problems surrounding the prohibition of prayer for the lifting of pestilence to five key issues:

First: If the plague is a mercy, how can one ask for it to be lifted?

Second: The one who is patient during plague is rewarded in the hereafter as if he were a martyr. In this way, is seeking that the plague be lifted equivalent to loathing this abundant heavenly reward?

Third: Believing in the Divine decree requires believing that only what is written for a person afflicts him. Is seeking to lift something that God has already decreed ineffective? Is it impossible?

Fourth: Given that the prohibition of fleeing from the plague has been established, is seeking that it be lifted a kind of fleeing?

Fifth: Given that the Prophet made a prayer for plague for his community, does seeking that it be lifted amount to opposing to him?

Al-Millawī responded to these questions in two parts—in general terms and in more detail. At a general level, al-Millawī argued that the legitimacy of performing prayer to lift pestilence is well established. Forbidding such a practice can only be accepted through a clear command prohibiting it; one that overturns its establishment. He further argued that the establishment of its religious legitimacy is obtained through evidence: One of them is praying for the healing of the sick. Another is praying for protection; another is seeking treatment, and he cites the hadiths that address these. Among these is ʿĀʾisha's hadith, recorded by Ibn al-Sunnī:

> The Prophet used to bless the land that he wanted to enter with the following prayer: "O God, I ask You for the good of this land, and the good of what is collected in it. I seek refuge in You from its evil and the evil of that which is gathered in it. O God, grant us its good harvest, protect us from its pestilence, endear us to its people, and endear the righteous among its people to us."[1]

At a more detailed level, I will now describe al-Millawī's rebuttal to the position that one should not pray for the lifting of the plague, point by point. Al-Millawī argued that the fact that the plague is a mercy does not negate asking God to lift the plague, because mercy is one thing and the plague's effect or cause is another thing. Effects and causes are of different levels. Perhaps the way that it works is that one seeks from God that which is a higher level of mercy than the plague.

As for the issue of the plague leading to martyrdom? Al-Millawī argued that martyrdom can be obtained by the one who withstands the plague patiently, putting trust in God, and being content with its occurrence even if it were to strike him, regardless of whether he prays for it to be lifted or not. For such a person, the act of seeking God alone and taking refuge in Him is desirable and recommended. The nature of the plague is that it is like meeting the enemy on the battlefield. Asking God for good health, free of the plague, has been religiously established, as has patience if the encounter with the plague occurs thereafter. Thus, what behooves him is not to wish for the plague, but to ask God for good health and to be free of it. If God decrees that the plague strike him, it behooves him to endure it patiently and be hopeful of heavenly reward for being afflicted by it.

In my view, these points are strengthened by what we have presented earlier concerning the fact that the plague results from the pricks of our enemies among the jinn. It is also strengthened by the fact that it is sufficient to comply with the following commands: to be patient when the plague occurs; to refrain from fleeing to another land to escape it; and to seek deliverance from it, without fretting or discontent.

This does not conflict with a slave asking his Lord for good health free of the plague, nor does it contradict believing in the Divine decree, because it is possible that God made the beseecher's prayer a cause for good health, free of the plague. It is also possible that God appoints for him the martyr's reward due to a person's patience and well-being free from the plague due to a person's prayer—each of these is from God's grace and mercy.

Seeking protection from many things has already been established, such that one who experiences them can become a martyr. Abū Dāwūd recorded that the Prophet used to pray:

> "O God, I seek refuge in You from destruction. I seek refuge in You from annihilation, and I seek refuge in You from drowning and burning, and I seek refuge in You from dying as a result of a bite."[2]

As for the fact that the plague is a thing decreed by God, al-Millawī noted that this is right and true. But this does not entail the prohibition of making supplications. In fact, such a prohibition would be a form of abandoning good deeds by merely submitting to what God has decreed. Taken to its logical conclusion, a prohibition of making supplications would require abandoning all the courses of action that result in different grades of eternal happiness, and it would be contrary to what God praised in the verse "those who pray to their Lord in the morning and the evening."[3] In addition, there is a hadith from the Prophet:

> "Do not hold back when supplicating to God. No one has ever been destroyed in light of his supplication."[4]

The Prophet also said:

> "The only way the Divine decree is reversed is through supplication."[5]

ʿĀʾisha also said the Prophet said:

> "It is not sufficient to merely fear the Divine decree, because supplication to God benefits the person for whom trials are

> sent and not sent. The tribulation sent by God comes down and encounters a supplication, and there is thereby a struggle between the two."[6]

In this way, the tribulation sent by God is diverted by the supplication, just as the spear is repelled by a shield. It is not a condition of believing in the Divine decree that one bear a spear while not protecting oneself with a shield.

The argument that supplication has elements that make it a type of fleeing is, according to al-Millawī, incoherent. For the meaning behind the prohibition from fleeing is that one not try to overcome the Divine decree through strength, power, and trickery. If they did, they would share a characteristic with those who "thought that their strongholds would protect them against God."[7] Supplication is the opposite of that. It is a recognition of the worshipper's lack of strength and cunning, along with the modesty and humility it entails, which do not contradict the acceptance of God's command and trust in His decree.

As for the Prophet praying for the plague to strike his community, does praying for it to be lifted amount to opposing to him?

Al-Millāwī's answer to that is that praying for the plague's cessation supports him, in that it is a plea to God to lift the hardship from his community. This does not deny his statement, "O God, give us the plague!" because this is not a request for it. Rather, its meaning is that God did not give non-believers an opportunity against them when the choice between the sword and the plague was presented to the Prophet, and that a disease sent from heaven would be sufficient for their destruction while preserving their honor. The plague was not sought by the Prophet for intrinsic reasons, neither in the first place nor the second. Rather, the intent was the preservation of a Muslim's honor, a repulsion of those who disbelieve through their rage, and a purification of the believers from the blood of their brothers.

Everything in the rebuttal that al-Millawī wrote is valid except for this last part of the hadith concerning the Prophet asking God to strike his community. The correct interpretation is that it is established as a clear request to God, as was clarified earlier in the third chapter.[8]

I would add, in sum, that the Prophet's prayer for his community to be afflicted by the plague does not require him to refrain from praying for its lifting when it occurs. The Prophet's request for it to occur is, in reality, asking for it to occur to someone, causing them to die at the end of their appointed lifetime, so they obtain the status of martyrdom through one of two ways—by the sword or the plague. His prayer for the plague to be lifted is in reality just asking that the plague not occur in a widespread way, killing a large number in a small amount of time, causing the desolation of most of the land, the loss of many livelihoods, and giving opportunity for the religion's enemies to rejoice at its expense. All of these are things for which the learned person does not refrain from praying.

The sense in which the plague is a calamity comes from the fact that it strikes a large number in a small period of time, as opposed to death, which occurs to one person at a time. The sense in which the plague is a mercy—and the fact that the one who dies from the plague is a martyr—does not contradict the fact that it is a calamity. This is the case in the same way that an enemy entering Muslim lands does not prevent one from praying for the safety of the Muslims and victory over their enemies, even as one who dies at the hands of the enemy is at that moment definitely a martyr. Al-Subkī inclined toward this answer. Then he said:

> This response applies insofar as the supplication is for lifting the plague in absolute terms from the people of a land. As for praying that the plague not occur to a specific person or oneself, it is not clear to me that there is something problematic in that. It is as if he is asking that the disease not descend upon him in particular. It is as if he said, "Do not give this unjust person power over me."
>
> The Prophet made a prayer for Anas to have long life, and the report of it has been established in the *Authentic Hadith*, in which the permissibility of praying for long life is quite clear. The same conclusion is taken from God's saying, "Ask your Sustainer to forgive you your sins, and then

turn toward Him in repentance—whereupon He will grant you a goodly enjoyment of life in this world until a term set by Him is fulfilled."[9] The same idea is found in other places.

PRAYING TO LIVE LONGER

The assumption that it is permissible or even recommended for one to pray for a long life is limited to praying for one who would benefit Muslims with their extended life. If the benefit of their long life would be limited to just themselves, then it is of a lower level than the former kind of prayer. Other than these two cases, such prayers for the lengthening of a life are disapproved and they are prohibited in situations that run counter to these two cases. Even in ordinary circumstances, some have said that no one should love what Satan loves, and he loves the lengthening of lives. But the truth is that the ruling depends on the specific circumstances. God knows best.

The religious scholars hold the view that the length of one's life neither increases nor decreases. But the benefit of prayer can be imagined in the following way: it is possible that God has determined Zayd's life to last thirty years, but if he prays for a longer life, then it is forty. Either way, one of the two will occur. This applies to all types of supplication—and if this is not the case, then there is no benefit in supplication, because all things are determined by God, the Exalted, may His power be glorified.

Al-Subkī held the following view:

> Muʿādh's prayer was not for God to lift the pestilence from the Muslims, but rather to seek it for himself, so he could obtain the status of a martyr.

In my opinion, Muʿādh's prayer was so that he might die having performed the purest of his deeds and undertaken jihād before the occurrence of the civil war, just as more than one of the Companions wished for themselves and which they explicitly stated as the reason for their desire. An example of this is recorded by Aḥmad, who cites ʿAlīm al-Kindī, who said:

> We were sitting on the terrace, and one of the Companions of the Prophet was with us. The people were leaving from the plague, and al-Ghifārī said, "Plague, take me!—Plague, take me!—Plague, take me!"
>
> ʿAlīm asked him, "Why are you saying this? Did not God's Messenger say: 'Let not one of you desire death, for it terminates one's deeds and he will not be brought back, so he should seek God's favor now. . . .'"
>
> Then ʿAlīm added: "I also heard God's Messenger saying: 'Six things hasten my community's demise: the rule of the foolish, having too many armed guards, judicial corruption. . . .'"[10]

In another version, al-Ṭabarānī cites Zādhān:

> I was on a terrace with one of the Companions of the Prophet named ʿAbbās or Ibn ʿAbbās, and he saw people hauling things away.
>
> He asked: "What's going on with those people?"
>
> He was told: "They are fleeing from the plague."
>
> And then he mentioned the hadith about the six things that hasten their demise.[11]

There are many beneficial points in this hadith: that one of the Companions censures people who flee from the plague; the permissibility of wishing for death out of fear of civil war; and the permissibility of the bearing of harm mentioned in the hadith over another worldly harm, but not over an otherworldly harm. But God knows best.[12]

As for the position that prohibits making supplications of any kind, we have already seen the response to it. In sum, it is not prohibited because there is no element in it that is prohibited. In fact, the Prophet has said, "But your recovery is more pleasing to me."

The best interpretation is that praying for recovery from

the plague or for the plague to be lifted differs according to the condition of the afflicted person in question. The one whose faith is certain and relies fully in God, his station is the highest. He trusts in God with his affairs and is saved, and he knows that what has stricken him is not because of his errors, and his errors were not caused by what has stricken him. If he is healthy, he is grateful; and if he is not healthy, then he is patient. He may even ascend to another level and seek martyrdom, as occurred with more than one among the Companions and the righteous ancestors.

Al-Jaṣṣās interpreted Abū ʿUbayda's actions in this light when he refused to leave Syria. It is for this reason that Muʿādh asked that he be given an abundant share of heavenly reward. Similarly, ʿUmar said: "O God, grant me martyrdom in Your path!"

One who does not reach this level, but accepts and comes to terms with it, does what has been established in Muslim's *Authentic Hadith* from Anas: that the Prophet commanded the Companions whose illness had become severe to make the following prayer:

> O God, allow me to live as long as life is better for me, and cause me to die when death is better for me.

If one fears that one's religion will succumb to temptation, and so prefers the continuation of an affliction over healing so that his religion may be safeguarded—he is rewarded for his intention, similar to what is recorded about ʿAbbās and ʿAwf. But it is permissible for someone who is not so inclined to seek that his Lord heal him from sickness. This is permitted on the condition that he is mindful that there is nothing that subverts what God has decreed, God is the one who determines that his prayer for healing is a cause for his healing and that this is not because God's decree was subverted through trickery. In this matter, there is no difference between those afflicted by either a severe fever, the plague, or any other sickness.

The hadith on the seventy thousand that shall enter heaven without suffering a Divine reckoning will provide guidance on this matter. Those seventy thousand are the ones who "do not practice sorcery, nor cauterize, nor invoke evil omens, and who rely entirely on their Lord." Al-Bukhārī and Muslim record this, along with other hadiths on the permissibility of seeking protection through the invocation of certain scriptural passages and seeking treatment and things of that nature.[13] Making supplication to lift the affliction is not forbidden, nor does it oppose that which God has decreed just because of the principle that God has decreed it.

As for making the supplication in congregation, as is the practice of performing the prayer for rain, it is a heretical practice that was fabricated during the Great Plague of the year 749 (1348) in Damascus. I read in al-Manbijī's collection that in the year 764 (1363), when the plague occurred in Damascus, someone gathered the people together in one place, an event he censured, and that they started praying, crying, and screaming. He noted that this also happened in 740 (1340): The common people and most of the country's leaders went out to the desert, prayed, and sought help from God. But the plague increased after the event and spread, when it had been much lighter before their prayer.

I would add that such a gathering in the desert occurred in our own time, when the plague first appeared in Cairo on the 27th of Rabīʿ II in the year 833 (1430). The number of people who died from the plague was less than forty. But then the people went out to the desert on the 4th of Jumādā I, after one of them called on people to fast for three days, just as they do in the ritual for praying for rain. They prayed in congregation and stood for an hour, then returned. By the end of the month, the number of those dying each day in Cairo was above one thousand and only continued to increase from there.

People have asked for legal opinions on the question of whether it was permissible to perform a ritual gathering in the desert to respond to the plague as if it were a drought. One of the people has delivered a legal opinion stating that it is authorized in the law, and he bases his legal opinion on the general sense of the reports about making supplication. Another scholar relied on the fact that it occurred in the time of Malik al-

Mu'ayyad and a group of scholars attended it without disapproving it, and that it fulfilled its purpose.

Another group of religious scholars delivered a legal opinion that refraining from such a practice is better, because of the fear of social disorder in it, regardless of whether it works or not. If it works, no one sees the danger of calling for it. But if it does not work, then the religious scholars, the pious, and the preachers are viewed in a bad light.

I incline toward this view in my own response but would add the following: If it is, in fact, authorized by the law, then the pious early generations would have known it, as would the religious scholars of the cities in the empires of past eras and their followers. But there survives no record, nor any report preserved by the hadith scholars, nor a jurist's interpretation of the law documenting such a practice.

The specific phrasing of prayers and the attributes of the one making the prayer have particular characteristics and secrets that are unique to each circumstance associated with it. So the accepted principle in cases like this is to follow scripture, without drawing on analogies to justify a novel practice. An example of this is what is recorded about what to do when experiencing fear from a solar eclipse. The recommended action has a specific form that is different from what is recorded about what to do when experiencing fear of droughts or what to do when experiencing hardship from things such as famine or diseases. Some hold that the qunūt is appropriate for the latter, which is different from the prayer responding to droughts and seeking rain. The one who uses this for that and that for this is one who has illegitimately added something new that does not belong to the commands of religion, and so it is rejected. Al-Shāfiʿī, may God have mercy on him, wrote that there is no qunūt for seeking rain, which strengthens what I have said here. But God knows best.

This is one of the reasons that caused me to draft this book, which I did after I collected most of the hadiths and some of the discussion on them in the year 819 (1416), when I refused to go out to the desert at that time. Nor was I present in the company of al-Malik al-Muʾayyad, because of the issue above, even though I had a special relationship with him. What happened at that gathering is what I imagined—using the prayer for rain to seek protection from the plague—and what was said was said. There is neither power nor might except with God, the most High, the Glorious.

One of the officials associated with al-Ṣalāḥ al-Sulṭān al-Ashraf gave a command, relying on a dream that he had, in which he was told that he should command the preachers, muezzins, teachers, and storytellers to finish their supplications with the following verse: "Our Lord, protect us from the torment, for we are believers."[14]

I was asked about this and responded by saying that the verse ought to be replaced with the following: "Our Lord, we have transgressed against ourselves."[15] My basis for that is that the profession of the content of this verse occurs as a gift to Adam, after which God, the Exalted, accepted his repentance and had mercy on him. Whereas the other verse is God's quotation of the disbelievers, which he follows up with a rejection of them. The verse that I have mentioned is more appropriate in this circumstance, by this measure and others.

Then I found, in Ibn Abī al-Dunyā's work, that when an earthquake occurred during his time, the caliph ʿUmar ibn ʿAbd al-Azīz wrote the following to all of the cities in the empire: that they should congregate for prayer at a specific time, and that those who had some wealth should give it away in charity, for God, the Exalted, says: "The one who purifies succeeds; and the one who remembers God's name and prays."[16] Moreover, he wrote that they proclaim the same thing as what Adam said: "Our Lord, we have transgressed against ourselves."[17]

This is the extent of the reports of the pious predecessors that has reached us, but nothing has reached us from the time of the Companions and the Successors saying that they offered congregational prayers asking for rain in this way. The exception is what happened in the year 49 (669): They offered a congregational prayer, made supplications, then returned, and the problem only got worse. Those who attempted did not obtain their desired purpose. The exact thing happened eighty-five years later.

We have already seen the story of ʿUmar ibn ʿAbd al-ʿAzīz's command to give things away in charity and to make supplication with the Qur'anic verse, "Our Lord, we have transgressed against ourselves." This is the oldest report I have found on the issue at hand, and it was mentioned with respect to earthquakes, and it is not impossible that one does something similar with respect to the plague. The element of fear is the uniting element between the two cases.

It has been said that al-Subkī wrote the following to his son Abū Ḥāmid on the plague in the year 749 (1348):

> A pious man had seen the Prophet in a dream in the Umayyad Friday Mosque. There were people around asking him to lift the pestilence and he responded, saying: "Loving One! Loving One! Possessor of the majestic throne! Creator and Resurrector! Accomplisher of all that He wills! I ask You through the light of Your countenance, which fills the pillars of Your throne, through Your power, which You deployed over Your creation, through Your mercy, which encompasses each thing, lift this pestilence that is upon us."

This supplication has come down regarding the story of the trader and the thief. The occurrence of the dream mentioned above is far-fetched, but it is possible.

In addition to this is what Ibn Abī Ḥajala recorded in a volume he put together on the reciting of blessings for the Prophet, in which he noted some things about the plague. He said: "It has spread to Cairo," by which he meant in the year 764 (1363). He continued: "When the plague became widespread in a given quarter, some pious folk saw the Prophet in a dream and complained to him of their condition. He ordered them to make this supplication:

> O God, we seek refuge in You from the sword and the plague, and the great afflictions upon our souls, wealth, family, and offspring. Allahu Akbar! Allahu Akbar! God is

> greater than that which we fear and of which we are afraid. Allahu Akbar! Allahu Akbar! God is great, the One who counts our sins and then forgives them. Allahu Akbar! Allahu Akbar! Allahu Akbar! May peace and blessings be upon our Master, Muhammad, and upon his family. Allahu Akbar! Allahu Akbar! Allahu Akbar! O God, just as You have accepted the intercession of our Prophet on our behalf, and granted us respite, and given us long lives in our homes, do not destroy us for our sins—Most Merciful of those who show mercy!

In my opinion, the validity of the opening part of this prayer is unlikely, because it conflicts with what we know about how the Prophet prayed for his community on this issue. Can one imagine that he would command them to seek protection from precisely that which he prayed for on behalf of them? But God knows best.

The littérateur Ibn Abī Ḥajala, in a volume he put together on the plague, mentions that one of the pious told him that the greatest defense against the plague and other severe afflictions is praying for God to bless the Prophet. He mentioned this to the Shaykh Shams al-Dīn ibn Khaṭīb Yabrūd, who confirmed its correctness and cited Ubayy ibn Kaʿb's hadith as proof:

> A man said to the Prophet: "May I make half of my prayer for you?"
>
> The Prophet replied: "If so, then your aspiration will suffice for you, and God will forgive your sins."

Al-Ḥākim records it and deems it to be authentic. Its isnad is strong. But God knows best.

THE WORDING OF THE QUNŪT PRAYERS DURING CALAMITIES

I was not able to find anything in the books of the jurists about the specific wording of the prayers they would recite during the qunūt for calamities. What is apparent is that they would delegate that practice to the understanding of the listener—that he would make a prayer that is appropriate to each calamity.

Al-Zarkashī remarked that one of the pious ancestors used to make this supplication after performing his daily prayers:

> "O God, we seek refuge in you from severe affliction, with respect to ourselves, family, property, and offspring."[18]

5.2

Is Widespread Plague Considered a Life-Threatening Situation for Legal Purposes?

Al-Subkī wrote:

> When plague emerges in a land, my colleagues are divided into two camps over whether it should be treated as life-threatening. Both views apply in cases when death has become widespread in an area. The more valid of the two opinions, according to al-Baghawī, is that it is, in fact, life-threatening from a legal standpoint. Al-Juwaynī attributes the view to al-Shāfiʿī, based on express record; but al-Māwardī concluded that the opposite was true in his work the *Encyclopedia*.[19]

As I see it, it is the preferred view of most Iraqi jurists, and al-Bandanījī's statement shows that he is one of them insofar as he quotes al-Shāfiʿī's view, may God have mercy on him, as saying: "The plague is life-threatening, until it disappears; this means that when the plague afflicts a particular person, it is considered life-threatening, until it leaves him." But, in fact, al-Shāfiʿī's statements are ambiguous and support both views, and do not explicitly favor one or the other.

The difference of opinions in this case is similar to the differences regarding a person who crosses paths with a lion or someone who finds himself in a building that catches fire. It is uncontroversial that he is in a life-threatening condition if the lion seizes him or the fire reaches a part of his body. But before that happens, there is a disagreement over whether the condition is life-threatening or not.

The upshot of the difference of opinion becomes apparent when we consider the issue of the restrictions on gratuitous property transactions placed on one in this condition. The legal scholar who enforces the restriction only on one afflicted by the disease allows one who is not personally afflicted by the plague full access to all of his wealth, even if he lives in an area afflicted by the plague. Meanwhile, the legal scholar who categorizes an otherwise healthy person as facing a life-threatening illness when the plague merely appears in a given area limits property transactions to a third of his wealth until the plague dissipates. If the person in question dies, the one-third restriction on valid property transactions remains in force. If he does not die, then it becomes apparent that he was not, in fact, in a life-threatening situation, as is the case in all types of life-threatening illnesses.

Al-Juwaynī's statement in his work *The Endpoint* is:

> Al-Shāfiʿī explicitly stated that if someone lives in a region in which the plague has reached and becomes widespread, then whoever is a resident there is considered to be in a life-threatening situation, even if he never falls ill with the plague.[20]

Qāḍī al-Ḥusayn offered the following evidence for why everyone in the plague-affected region should be considered as suffering from a life-threatening illness: the Prophet forbade leaving a region in which the plague occurs. He argues, based on this evidence, that when the plague occurs in a country, it afflicts all the inhabitants. But this argument is not obvious. After all, if it were the case, the restriction on gratuitous transfers of property would remain in force for those who left such a region for reasons other than fleeing the plague, in which case he would only be allowed to give away a third of his wealth; but I do not reckon that anyone holds this view.

Al-Zarkashī tried to resolve this dispute by saying that the two views apply to two different situations. The view that it is life-threatening holds when the plague appears in situations in which it becomes so widespread and lasts only a few days but kills most of the inhabitants of the town—with corpses rotting in their homes, with their doors firmly shut because no one is able to bury them, as the conditions in extreme plague have been described.* The view that it is not a life-threatening illness applies in cases where, when it occurs and spreads, death proliferates gradually, and it lasts an extended period of time, as has occurred regularly in recent times. In my view, this is a useful distinction.

Related to this is a situation of spread only among a subsection of the city's population—for example, if it spreads only among its slaves and children but not the men and the aged, for whom it is rare. This situation strengthens the view that, in this case, it is not a life-threatening condition for an area, but God knows best.

Al-Manbijī cites two views from Aḥmad. He said:

> Aḥmad was asked about the permissibility of giving away wealth during the plague, or while being out at sea, or while being on a military campaign, and he replied that "it is valid only up to a third of his wealth. Widespread plague is like being out at sea, and one afflicted by the plague is like one whose ship has broken up." In a second narration of Aḥmad's view, he holds that "gratuitous transactions are valid with-

*This is likely depicting what we would now describe as the pneumatic form of the plague, which spread and killed with much greater speed than the bubonic form.

out restriction," meaning until one is actually afflicted by the plague.[21]

The basis for the first view is that death is expected in those cases, like one on the front lines of battle. He worries that he will suffer what those around him have suffered because he sees death seize his neighbors or even seize someone in his own home, so his own life is at great risk.

The basis for the second view is that the power of a person of sound health to give gifts is valid without limitation. We have already refuted the medical experts' claim that the plague originates in corrupt air and thereby affects anyone who breathes it in. The existence of a general cause is not the same as the existence of a particular cause. Someone exposed to a specific cause is actually stricken by the disease, while one exposed to a general cause is not yet stricken by it. Accordingly, how can the law treat someone who expects a disease whose likely outcome is death the same as someone who expects death itself? I have not seen the Mālikīs or the Ḥanafīs address this.

In my understanding, the issue is reported in Mālikī books, and they have two different narrations regarding it. The better-supported view among them is that the unafflicted person living in a place threatened by plague is treated as someone in sound health. As for the Ḥanafīs, while they do not explicitly address this specific issue in their texts, their principles require them to categorize an unafflicted person in a plague-afflicted area in the same way the Mālikīs do. This is what a group of their scholars have told me. To sum up, the stronger view among the later Shāfiʿīs is the weaker view in the minds of most non-Shāfiʿī scholars. And God knows best.

One effect of classifying a person living amid a plague as facing a life-threatening illness is the following related disagreement: if one irrevocably divorces his wife and he subsequently dies while she is in her post-divorce waiting period, does she inherit from him, as in the old view, or not? There are other such subsidiary legal issues.

If we assume that one is suffering from a life-threatening

illness, then it is obvious that it is religiously praiseworthy for one to incline toward hope in recovery more than fear of demise or at least have equal amounts of both.

There is no doubt that acting promptly to rectify one's transgressions against others, repenting from sins and wrongdoings, and seeking forgiveness for interfering in things that ought not concern one are religiously praiseworthy acts. Nay, they are obligatory, in both sets of circumstances, and authorized by the law in all circumstances. It is just that they are all the more important in the case of the ill, even if the illness is not life-threatening, and in the case of a disease that threatens the health of the general public but not the individual. When the illness is life-threatening, then the obligatory character of these actions is even greater for the person suffering it; this is the case of one afflicted by the plague, but God knows best.

5.3

On What Physicians Advise to Protect Oneself against the Plague

A final conclusion arises from the view that prohibits entering a town struck by the plague: the practice of protecting oneself from a trial by plague. The religious legitimacy of seeking treatment is one of the proofs for following the advice of physicians to protect oneself during an epidemic. They advise eliminating excessive fluids from the body, minimizing eating, abstaining from exercise, spending time in the bathhouse, getting rest, and reducing the inhalation of contaminated air.

The master Avicenna clearly said that the first thing one must do in treating the plague is to make an incision in the buboes, if possible. Then one drains what is in them, without stopping until it congeals, drawing out its poison. If necessary, it can be sucked up using a cupping glass, if done so lightly. He also said:

> The plague may be treated by what compresses and cools, using a sponge soaked in vinegar and water or rose oil, apple oil, or myrtle oil. The plague-afflicted patient can also be treated through evacuations, such as through bloodletting, if he is able to bear it at the time. If not, one delays it if the humor has been extracted. Then he should proceed to preserve and strengthen the heart using cooling and perfuming agents, and provide drugs used to treat people with hot heart palpitations.

In my opinion, the physicians of our time and the preceding generation have neglected this regimen. The current consensus has forsaken this practice of treating the plague-afflicted patient with bloodletting, such that the absence of this practice has become so widespread and common that most physicians believe that treating plague patients through bloodletting is forbidden. This quotation from the master Avicenna contradicts what they prescribe, and reason supports him. As we already said, the plague-pricking stirs and agitates the existing blood in the body. The blood then moves to another place from there until its harm reaches the heart, which is fatal. For this reason, Avicenna, when he mentioned the treatment with making incisions and bloodletting, noted that it was necessary.

Avicenna mentions that a group of physicians cautioned against the healthy visiting those afflicted with the plague. Al-Subkī said, in response:

> In our opinion, the public should be prevented from mixing with the plague-stricken, such that they even stop visiting them. We say that if two knowledgeable, virtuous Muslim physicians, or someone who reaches that level, testify that there is harm caused when the healthy mix with the plague-stricken, then it is permissible to keep them from mixing.[22]

In my view, the notion that harm is caused by the healthy visiting the sick cannot be taken to be true, because the senses belie it. These plagues have recurred in the lands of Egypt and Syria to the point that few households have been spared from it. Yet one finds that someone is afflicted by it, and his family members and other members of the household—such as domestic servants or slaves—continue to live with him. Their mixing with him is significantly greater than the mixing of strangers and non-household members can ever be. Yet, many, nay, most members of the plague-stricken patient's household remain healthy. Whoever thinks that mixing causes harm is stubborn in holding such an opinion.

What we have discussed in terms of demonstrating the falsity of contagion relieves us of the need to rehash it here. Al-Subkī, God have mercy on him, proceeded to affirm the existence of contagion in reliance on nature's customary course. He further held that texts that deny contagion were simply intended to convey that the plague is not by its essential nature contagious.

Al-Qurṭubī, in his *Giver of Understanding*, has said:

> The idea of contagion is one of the false imaginings of the ignorant Arabs, because they used to believe that when a sick person met healthy people, he would make them sick. The Prophet negated this and invalidated it and vanquished their doubts with a single word, when he asked: "So then who infected the first?" Its meaning is: From where did mange come? From another camel that scratched it? This would require an infinite regress, which is logically impossible. Or from some cause other than camels? The one who caused the first itch is the one who caused the second, which is God, the Creator of everything and the One with power over all things. . . . Those who believe in the idea of contagion using specious reasoning are called naturalists. They hold that things affect one another, and they name the cause "nature."
>
> The Muʿtazila are the second group who hold this false premise, and they advance this notion with respect to the actions of animals. They hold that animals' capacity for action is the cause of the existence of the effect, and that they are the creators of their own acts, independent in originating them.
>
> These two groups rely on empirical observation to support their argument. Sometimes they label those who deny

> this as those who deny self-evident truths, but this is incorrect. The error is rooted in mistaking the perception of the senses for the perception of the intellect. That which they witness is only the effect of one thing in the proximity of another, which is the domain of the senses. As for causation, it is not perceived by the senses, but by the intellect. But God knows best.

In my view, the gist of the positions on the idea of contagion are four:

The first is the view of the disbelievers: the sick person infects others, and only by the disease's essential nature.

The second is an Islamic view, but it is not the preferred one: the sick person infects through a thing that God creates and places in that person, from which he cannot ever detach, except by way of a miracle of some sort, and only then would his condition change.

The third is that the sick person infects, not on account of the disease's essential nature, but through a customary chain of events that God puts into effect most times. This line of thinking is similar to the idea that He puts the customary chain of events into effect in the case of lighting a fire. But this can change if God wills, even as this change is rare in the customary chain of events.

The fourth is that the sick person does not ever transmit illness to others on account of the disease's essential nature. Rather, the sickness that occurs in him is the result of God's direct act of creation in him—glory be to Him, and may He be exalted. For this reason, you see many who have been afflicted by the disease and regarded as capable of transmitting it—yet when healthy people mix with the sick, the disease does not afflict the healthy in the slightest. You also see many who do not mix with the diseased person ever, yet the sickness afflicts them. All of this is because of what God ordained.

The last two positions are common. The one that is best supported is the last one, based on the spirit of the Prophet's saying: "There is no contagion"; and his response to those who affirmed the idea of contagion: "Then who infected the first?" But God, may He be glorified and exalted, knows best.

5.4

Select Hadiths on the Proper Conduct for Those Afflicted with the Plague and Other Illnesses

The first rule of conduct is asking God for health and protection from sickness. God, the Glorified, the Exalted, said in the Qur'an:

> Call on your Lord, openly, or in secret.[23]

And, the Prophet said to ʿAbbās:

> "Increase the supplicatory prayers for health."[24]

Ibn ʿUmar cites the Prophet:

> "God is not asked for anything more beloved to him than health."[25]

Abū Hurayra cites God's Messenger:

> "There is no supplication God's servant makes that is more excellent than the following: 'O God, I ask you for health in this life and the next.'"[26]

Abū Bakr al-Ṣiddīq cites the Prophet, who said:

> "The only thing the people have been given better than certain faith is health."[27]

From ʿUthmān ibn Abī al-ʿĀṣ, who said:

He complained to the Prophet about an ache in his body.

The Prophet told him, "Put your hand where you feel the pain in your body, and say 'in the name of God' three times, then say the following seven times: "I seek refuge in God and His Power from the evil I find and guard against."[28]

Asmāʾ bint Abū Bakr said:

There emerged a protrusion on my neck, and I became scared and told ʿĀʾisha. She said to me: "The Prophet gently removed it for me."

So I asked him about it.

He replied, "Put your hand on it, then say three times: 'In the name of God, repel the evil that I find and its devilry, by the supplication of your noble, blessed, and steadfast Prophet who is with you, in the name of God.'"

Then she said: "I said it, and it went away."[29]

Abū al-Dardāʾ said he heard God's Messenger say:

"Let him who complains about a problem or whose brother complains about a problem to him say the following so that he may recover: 'Our Lord, God, in heaven, manifest Your mercy on earth, and forgive us our sins and missteps. You are the Lord of the virtuous. Deliver to us a merciful act from Your mercy, and an act of healing upon this pain.'"

From Ibn ʿAbbās, who said:

God's Messenger used to teach us the following words in regard to aches and fever: "In the name of God, the Great, I seek refuge in God, the Mighty, from the evil of every howling pain and the fire's heat."[30]

The second rule of conduct is having patience with God's decree and being content with what He ordained. The following is a short explanation of this:

Ṣuhayb said that the Prophet said:

> "How happy is the believer's affair! Every circumstance is good for him; this is not for anyone but the believer. If good things come to him, he is grateful; and that is good for him. If hardship afflicts him, he is patient, and that is good for him."[31]

Sakhbara said that God's Messenger said:

> "One who is given is grateful. One who is tried is patient. One who does wrong seeks forgiveness. One who is wronged is forgiven."
>
> The Companions asked: "God's Messenger, what is his recompense?"
>
> He recited the Qur'anic verse: "Theirs is peace and they are rightly guided."[32]

Abū Hurayra said that God's Messenger said:

> "God puts to the test the one for whom He desires good."

From Muḥammad ibn Labīd, that God's Messenger said:

> "When . . . God loves a people, He tries them. The one who is patient, has patience; the one who gets anxious has anxiety."[33]

From Abū Hurayra, who said that God's Messenger said:

> "Each man has a station with God, which man cannot achieve through his actions alone. But God continues to try him with what man dislikes until He helps him reach it."[34]

The third rule of conduct is encouraging one to think well of God, the Glorified, the Exalted. This applies especially to the case of one with a life-threatening illness. For one in this case the advice is as follows. He should call to mind the following: he is but a contemptible thing in God's creations; God's mercy encompasses those many things greater than he; that God, the Exalted, has no need of punishing him; that he recognize his sins and shortcomings; that he firmly believe that actions and intercessions of only those that God permits for that issue will secure him forgiveness or pardon; and he should remember the Qur'anic verses and hadiths on the theme of hope.

Muʿtamir ibn Sulaymān said:

> My father, at the moment of his death, encouraged me to take advantage of the Law's dispensations so that I may meet God thinking well of Him.
>
> He then turned his entire focus to asking God to end his life with goodness and cause him to die professing belief in God's oneness.

Some of the best hadiths on thinking well of God are found in al-Bukhārī's *Authentic Hadith*:

Shaddād ibn Aws said the Prophet said:

> "The best way of seeking forgiveness is to say: 'O God, You are my Lord, there is no god but You. You created me and I am Your servant. I fulfill my duties to You and rely on Your promise to the best of my ability. I seek refuge in You from the evil I have done. I confess to You my sins, and I acknowledge Your blessings upon me. Forgive me, for none forgivves sins but You.'
>
> The one who says this when he wakes up enters heaven if he should die that day. The one who says this when he goes to sleep enters heaven if he should die that night."

Al-Tirmidhī records the following Prophetic hadith:

> "Whoever says, 'There is no god but God, God is the Greatest, there is no god but God alone, without partner, to whom belongs sovereignty and praise, there is no god but

God, and there is no power but with God,'—the one who recites this while sick, then passes away—the fire will not touch him."[35]

The fourth rule of conduct is to visit the sick, which has merits. Abū Hurayra said that God's Messenger said:

"When one visits a sick person, a caller calls out from the sky: may you be happy and may your walking be blessed, and may you be awarded a lofty station in heaven."[36]

ʿĀʾisha said:

When a person complained about some issue with his health, whether it be an ulcer or a wound, the Prophet would point his finger at the earth, and say: "In the name of God, this dust of our land, mixed with our spittle, heals our sick by our Lord's permission."[37]

Abū Saʿīd al-Khudrī said:

Gabriel came to the Prophet and said, "Muhammad, have you complained of an issue with your health?"

"Yes," the Prophet replied.

Gabriel said: "In God's name, I offer a prayer to protect you from everything that harms you, whether it be the evil of each soul, or an evil eye. May God heal you."[38]

Abū Umāma said that God's Messenger said:

"The proper way to visit the sick is that you should put your hand on his face or hand and ask him how he is."[39]

Al-Aṣbagh ibn Nubāta said:

I entered with ʿAlī ibn Abī Ṭālib into al-Ḥasan ibn ʿAlī's presence, to visit him.

ʿAlī asked him: "How have you been, son of God's Messenger?"

Al-Ḥasan replied: "I have recovered."

ʿAlī replied, "May that be the case, God willing!"[40]

Ibn ʿAbbās said:

ʿAlī left God's Messenger's presence. The people asked him: "Father of al-Ḥasan, how is God's Messenger doing?"

He replied, "May God be praised, he has recovered."[41]

EPILOGUE

A RECORD OF PLAGUES

Plagues in the Time of Islam

The plagues during the time of Islam were briefly mentioned by al-Madāʾinī, then Ibn Abī al-Dunyā and Ibn Qutayba. One later scholar who lived in our time expanded upon these accounts, enumerating them in nearly forty sections. However, most of it deals with designating catastrophes in which many perished, such as a famine after a drought, or a fever with chills, or a fatal catarrh. I have summarized these events here, especially if I determined there was a great mortality brought about by the plague.

Five great plagues were well-known during the time of Islam,* according to the historian Abū al-Ḥasan al-Madāʾinī:

> The Plague of Sheroe,† which occurred in the city of Madāʾin‡ during the lifetime of God's Messenger; the Plague of ʿAmwās,§ which struck in Damascus during the time of ʿUmar, in which twenty-five thousand died; the Jārif Plague,¶ which struck in the year 69 (688); the Girls' Plague, which struck in the year 87 (706); and the Plague in Egypt during the year 66 (685).[1]
>
> ʿAbd al-ʿAzīz ibn Marwān fled Egypt in that year—he was the governor at the time—to a village he had and

*All dates listed here should be considered approximate; death counts should also be regarded as an estimation.

†A Sassanian king also known as Kavad II, who died of the plague in 628.

‡Madāʾin was an ancient city near the Sassanian capital of Ctesiphon, now located in modern Iraq.

§A locale near Jerusalem.

¶Called so for its lethal spread across Iraq.

settled there. A messenger from his brother, the Caliph ʿAbd al-Malik, traveled there to fetch him.

"What is your name?" ʿAbd al-ʿAzīz asked the courier.

The courier replied, "Ṭālib ibn Mudrik."

ʿAbd al-ʿAzīz groaned with disease and said: "I cannot see myself returning to Cairo." So ʿAbd al-ʿAzīz died in that village.

Add to this list the plague in which Ziyād ibn Abīhi died,* and the Sweeping Plague, though there is a disagreement about the year it took place. Some say it took place in the year 69 (688). Some say 72, others say 70 (691 or 689). Still others say it happened in some other year.

The Girls' Plague, which struck in the year 87 (706), was named so on account of the number of young women who died in it.

There was also the Notables' Plague, which struck when al-Ḥajjāj ibn Yūsuf was in Wāsiṭ, until it was said: "Let there be no more plague and al-Ḥajjāj!"†

The Plague of ʿAdī ibn Arṭāt, the governor of Baṣra, struck in the year 100 (718).

Syria saw one in 107 (725) and then again in 115 (733).

The Plague of Salim ibn Qutayba struck in the year 131 (748). Al-Madāʾinī said: "It was in Baṣra during the month of Rajab, and it hit hardest during Ramadan and let up during the month of Shawwāl. At its height, there were a thousand funerals a day."

All of this happened during the Umayyad Dynasty. But some historians note that the plagues were continuous in Syria during the time of the Umayyads; for this reason the Umayyad caliphs fled to the desert when the plagues started. Hishām ibn

---

*A governor of Iraq, who died around the year 53/673 of the Islamic Calendar.

†Al-Ḥajjāj was a controversial governor of Iraq during the Umayyad period; the author is making a parallel between the tragedy brought about by both the plague and the politics of the time. See Michael Dols, "Plague in Early Islamic History," *Journal of the American Oriental Society*, 94:3 (1974): 379.

ʿAbd al-Malik took up residence in a palace in Ruṣāfa, an ancient Roman outpost.

The Plague eased during the Abbasid Dynasty. This story is often told:

> One of the Abbasid commanders in Syria delivered a speech saying: "Praise be to God, who has dispelled the plague upon you ever since we came to rule over you."
>
> An audacious person in the audience then stood up and heckled: "God is more just than to impose your rule upon us at the same time as the plague!"

During the Abbasid Dynasty, a plague struck Rayy in the year 134 (751). It struck in Baghdad in the year 146 (763).

It struck Baṣra in the year 221 (836), which the book *The Well-Ordered* records, stating: "Many people died. There was even one person who had seven children, all of whom died in a single day."

The plague struck Iraq in the year 249 (863), and again in the year 301 (913). The plague struck Isfahan in the year 324 (935) and again in the year 346 (957). Death would pile up with little warning, to the point that if a judge dressed in his robes to go to court and was then struck by plague, he would die while still wearing one of his slippers.

The plague struck Baṣra in the year 406 (1015).

There was a Great Plague in the lands of India and Persia in the year 423 (1032). There was much death in Ghaznā, Khurāsān, Jurjān, Rayy, Isfahan, and the environs of al-Jabal to Ḥulwān. It spread to Mosul. At that point, it was said that the plague had brought Isfahan forty-one thousand funerals. It then spread to Baghdad.

Then the plague struck Shīrāz in the year 425 (1033). It reached the point that homes containing families who had died were boarded up because of the lack of people to properly prepare them for burial.

Then it spread to Wāsiṭ, Ahwāz, Baṣra, and Baghdad. At its height, many multitudes were dying. It was said that over the course of a few days, seventy thousand had died.

The plague struck Mosul, al-Jazīra, and Baghdad in the year 439 (1047). In Mosul, they performed the funeral prayer over four hundred souls at one time, and the death count reached three hundred thousand people.

The plague reached the Ḥijāz and Yemen in the year 452 (1060). At that time, many villages were destroyed, and no one lived there after that time. Anyone who entered there would perish within the hour.

Then the plague reached Egypt in the year 455 (1063), where people died of it over the course of ten months; every day a thousand souls were taken.

Sibṭ ibn al-Jawzī records in *The Mirror* for the year of 449 (1057) that a letter from Bukhārā arrived in the month of Jumādā II (August), noting that the people there faced utter annihilation the likes of which had never been seen or heard. At that time, eighteen thousand people left the region in a single day. Those who died were trapped there, and they numbered 1,650,000.

Then the disease reached Azerbaijan, then Ahwāz, then Wāsiṭ, then Baṣra. There reached a point where people were digging pits and threw in twenty or thirty corpses at a time.

It then spread to Balkh and Samarqand, and every day six thousand or more died. People worked day and night to wash, wrap, and bury the bodies. Among them was one whose heart cleaved, spouting out its blood, which then would emerge as a drop from the person's mouth, and then he would gurgle while dying. Sometimes a maggot would come out of his mouth without his realizing what it was, and he would then die.

More than two thousand households in the city shut down, and not a single person remained in them. The people repented, gave alms, attached themselves to the mosques, and devoted themselves to reciting the Qur'an. They threw out their wines and destroyed their musical instruments. If it so happened that a house had wine, its family would pass away in a single night; or if a man had sex unlawfully with a woman, both would die together.

One group entered a house, and they found a man grappling with death; he pointed to his cabinet, and there was a jug of wine. They poured it out, but still his hour came. He was a teacher of nine hundred children, and not one of them survived.

In Samarqand alone, 236,000 died from the 10th of Shawwāl until the end of the month of Dhū al-Qaʿda (December to January). This plague first began in Turkistan, then it went to Kāshghar and Farghāna, then it entered Samarqand. It did not enter Balkh or go beyond the Oxus River. At one point, a group left Bukhārā for Balkh and made camp at a fort, and all of them died just outside of Balkh.

Most of the dead were women, babies, children, teenagers, and young adults, rather than the middle-aged. More middle-aged numbered among the dead than elderly, and more of the common people died than the class of military officers. In sum, only a few of the military, authorities, or aged died.

The plague first struck in Syria and Egypt, then Baghdad, in 448 (1056), and the number of dead each day in Egypt reached ten thousand.

Then it spread to Egypt in the year 445 (1054) and continued until 446 (1055). It began in the spring and continued until the fall. Ibn Baṭlān remarked in a treatise that the Sultan buried eighty thousand dead that year.

One thousand died in Egypt each day in the year 455 (1063).

The plague struck Damascus in 469 (1076). From a population of approximately five hundred thousand, none but thirty thousand five hundred remained. Out of two hundred forty bakers, only two survived!

The plague struck Iraq again in the year 478 (1086), then became widespread around the world, such that the road was even closed to people living in travel outposts. Sibṭ ibn al-Jawzī related this in *The Mirror.*

The plague brought a great death to Baghdad in the year 575 (1180).

Then a great death came to Egypt in the year 597 (1201), but it was caused by some disease other than the plague.

Then a great plague struck Egypt in the year 633 (ca. 1236), and many of its people died during it.

Then came the Great Plague, in the year 749 (ca. 1348), which

Ibn al-Wardī, al-Ṣafadī, and Ibn Abī Ḥajala and others described, as we will see. No one in history has known anything like it. It spread across the earth from east to west; it even entered the holy city of Mecca.

Then the plague struck Cairo and Damascus in the year 764 (ca. 1363), but it was less severe than the Great Plague that preceded it.

The plague recurred in the year 770 (1369) in Damascus, then again in 781 (1380) in Cairo, and again in 791, 810, 819, 821 (1389, 1408, 1416, 1418), and again in the year that followed.

The plague struck yet again in the year 833 (1430). It was more widespread than all the plagues above combined, and deadlier than them. Nothing had occurred like it in Cairo or Egypt since the Great Plague of 749 (1349). It differed from the plagues of the past in numerous ways. For instance, the plague hit during the winter and disappeared during the spring. In the past, the plagues would occur during the springtime, only after winter had passed, and disappear at the beginning of the summer.

Another way in which it differed was that, during plagues of the past, most of those who died of the plague were usually delirious by the time of their passing. During this plague, by contrast, most of those who died did so fully aware and deeply distraught over their fate. They had certain knowledge of their impending death, and yet they could not benefit their souls, nor could their loved ones protect them from it.

Another way it differed was that there were numerous accounts from many people who suffered from the plague who reported heavenly visions, one after another. They beheld beautiful dreams that foretold all kinds of wonderful news. God be praised for that.

The beginning of that plague was from lands bordering Egypt on the lower terrestrial side. Then the plague entered Egypt proper. It approached Cairo from the coast, entering the city in the final part of the month of Rabīʿ II (January). The plague intensified from the middle of Jumādā I (February) to the middle of Jumādā II (March). It then declined from the first half of Jumādā II to the latter part of the month of Rajab (April). When the month of Shaʿbān (May) came, the plague was greatly diminished. It was lifted altogether after that. No one was added to the death register except those who would have normally died in an era that was free of plague.

Then the plague struck in the year 841 (1438) in the lands of Egypt beginning during Ramadan (March). By the end of the month, the death count reached a hundred, then another thousand were added to the death register during the month of Muḥarram of 842 (July 1438). More were added in the month of Ṣafar (August). It began to diminish on the 6th day of Ṣafar (July 29).[2]

Depictions of the Plague

Most of the depictions of the plague concern the Great Plague of the year 749 (1348). The best and most expert of those depictions is what my teacher Abū al-Yusr Aḥmad ibn ʿAbdullāh ibn al-Ṣāʾigh told me. He said that Shaykh Zayn al-Dīn ʿUmar ibn Muẓaffar ibn al-Wardī gave him permission in person to transmit this work of rhyming prose called "Tidings of the Plague."[3] It goes like this:

God is my surety, through every hardship. His oneness is all I require and all His servant needs. Bless Muhammad, grant him ease, may he intercede and keep us from this disease.

The Plague struck,
fear and death
followed.
For fifteen years,
he roved, then lingered,
in China,
in India and Sind,
far past the Oxus,
in the land of Uzbeks.

For fifteen years,
all were ensnared
by his dreaded hand.
None were spared:
in every stronghold, he found weakness.

Count them—
how many perished
in Persia, Rome, and Cyprus?
How many vanished
from Crimea to the land of Khitans?
In Cairo, he crept upon every creature
on whom he cast his eye—
for they are on this earth.

In Alexandria,
he stilled her draw-looms.
At her dār al-tirāz,
he spun,
like a slinking silkworm,
her spinners' fate.

Alexandria,
City of Pestilence,
a beast roars.
Patience—
even when only seven
of every seventy
remain.

To the highlands of Egypt,
he stormed and scourged.
To Cyrenaica,
to Gaza, Acre, and Ashkelon,
he scoured and shook.
In Jerusalem,
rock-hearted,
he seized those who fled

to that farthest mosque
beside the dome,
and paid the alms-tax with their souls,
returning what belonged
to One Alone. The Only One,
at this world's end, to open Mercy's door.

So he rushed
to the coast,
and thrashed his way
to Sidon, to Beirut,
he trapped, he ambushed.
His arrows pierced
Damascus,
and he sat, enthroned,
as his pustules slaughtered,
a thousand,
and a thousand more,
day upon day
upon days.
One Alone: Keep Damascus and her fragrant gardens safe,
snuff out this growing fire.

Allah!
Set Damascus straight.
Give her shelter.
Allah—
Her spirit will wither,
until she is slain,
by a bubo.

Mounting a stallion
to al-Mazza, to Barza,
he charged
to Baʿlbak, to Qāra.
A cry could be heard:
"Halt, let us weep,
for the sick of al-Nabak!"

From al-Jubba, to Shamsīn,
From Zabadānī to Ḥimṣ,
he robbed the sky of sun,
in a feverish downpour
he washed out
al-Ghasūla,
her coffins floating
to the banks of the Orontes River.
Ḥamā shivered, as he made himself at home.

Pestilence!
Ḥamā was once
a fortress.
You envelop her air
with your fetid breath,
and your kiss
upon her hills
is poisonous.

In Maʿarrat al-Nuʿmān,
he soothed:
"Hush hush—
Ḥamā's hurt
has quenched
my thirst."

He beheld the village of Maʿarra
as a heavenly nymph,
her coal-black eyes
alluring,
but her brow was battered
by abuse.
What can a plague do to a place
that tyranny thrust
to the ground?

He marched
upon Sarmīn and Fūʾah,

and rattled
Sunni and Shi'a.
He offered Antioch
an ample share,
before retreating,
whirling,
as a man
lost in flashes
of his beloved
in the campfire
embers.

He cooed
to Shayzar and al-Ḥārim,
"Calm—
you were in ashes
before I came,
and in ashes
you will be after I go.
Calm, calm—in time,
these ruins
will be rebuilt."

He snaked
through the jebels
and wadis
to ʿAzāz, to al-Bāb,
to Tal Bāshir, to Dhullil,
he pillaged, he plundered,
he brought them to their knees,
and plucked them from their keeps.

He pounced on Aleppo,
but he fell flat.
God eased
their burden.
No, I could not say
he grew,

like a plant,
with offshoots.

He slipped
into Alep.
They cried:
"It's war—on all humanity!"
I answered:
"A plague is a plague is a plague."

He preyed upon every house.
If one spat blood,
all spat blood
and in two nights—
maybe three—
were put underground.

I begged the Creator:
"Lift this piercing
plague!"
Someone spots
a drop of blood
and senses
the abyss.

Allah!
Dispel
this pestilence.
He acts
on Your orders!
Who can protect
us against this horror
other than You,
All Powerful?

God is greater
than this accursed disease

who pierces the mind
with madness,
who sharpens the spear-tip
he points at every medina.
I am aghast
at this spiked
and hated
thing.

How many a place did he enter!
With a torch he searched,
if those who dwelled there would not come,
he swore he would not leave.
His snake slithered
into Aleppo
spawning panic.
He was called
the Plague of Ansāb
the most dreadful
in the time of Islam,
the Great Death
the noble Muhammad
warned would come.

Aleppo,
Land of Suffering!
The pestilence has become
a vicious
serpent—
she kills
your people
with her
venomous
spit.
By God!
Her evil
is enough.

If you could have seen the elites of Aleppo
poring over arcane books of medicine,
where numerous remedies abounded.
They ate dried foods and citrus,
slathered themselves with Armenian mud,
brought their humors into balance,
scented their homes
with ambergris
camphor,
sedge and sandalwood,
adorned themselves with ruby rings,
and dined on onions, vinegar, and sardines.
In place of nourishing broth
and honeyed-fruits,
was citron, citron,
citron.

If you had seen Aleppo,
the caskets crawling
across every corner,
if you had heard
the sobs
and howls,
you would have fled,
abandoning
your homes.

The undertakers' wages rose,
their labor's sweat
was sweet.
But they played and preyed
upon their customers
like hustlers,
even as they turned
most of them away.
May their sweat turn sour.
May they go unrewarded.

The swindlers and the cheats
have turned silver-gray Aleppo
pitch-black in my eyes.
The coffin makers
have begun to dig
their own graves.

We ask for God's forgiveness
for those souls fallen to temptations.
This plague is part of His Trials and Tribulations.
We seek refuge from His Wrath and His Punishment.
We find shelter in His Healing and His Favor.

"*The corruption of the air ravages!*"
No. Rather,
the error of corruption savages.
How many a sin,
how many a wrong
do those who wail
make known!

The damned
people of Sīs
brought misery
and anger
to Islam
as they exulted
in this disease.
As if they were safe
from him—
as if they brokered a truce
with him—
as if they reigned triumphant
upon him—
as if, as if,
as if—
Oh Lord!

Do not allow us to be preyed upon
by those who disbelieve.

The city of Sīs.
like enemies of religion,
celebrate
what strikes us with grief.
So it is.
Before long,
God will deliver
this same sentence
upon them, a plague
upon a plague.

For those who believe,
the plague makes them martyrs,
the plague showers reward.
For those who disbelieve,
the plague punishes,
the plague's thunderclaps warn.
When a Muslim endures
his hardship with patience,
patience itself is worship.
"The plague-pierced are martyrs,"
thus spoke the Prophet.
This established tradition
is a law of martyrdom,
and a hidden wellspring
that delights the true believer.

A pretender may say:
"Contagion is the cause of this disaster!"
Reply: "No. Rather,
God has given and God has taken away."
If he insists on this illusion, ask, as our trusted Prophet once did:
"Then who caused the first infection?"
And if the plague takes
the rest of our family

but spares us,
this is the Will
of the One and Only.
Lord, God,
in You I seek
refuge
from the evil
of the Plague
of Ansāb.

His gunpowder bursts across nations,
and anyone watching the explosions is gripped
with reason-confounding fear.
He chases down those screaming in panic.
His flywheel spins,
no ransom,
no hoarded treasure
can be paid—
his flywheel
spins.

He breaks down the door
of a house, swearing,
"I have a warrant
for you and your family's arrest,
and will not leave
without taking you all."

And yet, there they are—
The Merits of the Plague:
freeing one from the desires of worldly gain,
perfecting one's deeds,
awakening one to forgotten obligations,
readying one for the final journey.

In plague-times,
one person begs another
to care for his children,

while another
bids farewells to his brothers.
One person betters his acts,
while another
prepares his burial shroud.
One person brokers peace
with his enemies,
while another
swells with generosity.
One person gives away
his property to God,
while another
emancipates
his slaves.
One person regains
his righteousness,
while another
finds
his
moral
compass.

~

This pestilence
delivers
a torrent,
a fire,
and in our time
there is no safeguard from him
other than God's Mercy, praise Him alone.

If we had not clung to the hadiths, we would have fled. So seek help from the Almighty God, who offers the greatest relief. O God, none before us have called on you as we do now to ward off this Plague and Pestilence. We will pray for its end and for our health to no one but You. O God, Lord

> of the Cleaving, we seek refuge in You from this Striking Rod. We beg You for Your Mercy, which is more expansive than our offenses, though they number the grains of sand. We beseech You, by the most generous intercessors, Muhammad, Prophet of Mercy, alleviate our deep distress. Protect us, God, shelter us from this Evil and Torment. Sublime Guardian, we are wholly dependent on You.

That is the best of what has been said on the plague—the most eloquent and elegant in terms of its expression and phrasing.

I read in the book of the Shaykh Shihāb al-Dīn Aḥmad ibn Yaḥyā ibn Abī Ḥajala,[4] who depicted the Great Plague:

> The plague
> spread throughout the land,
> decimated God's servants,
> crippled every mountain pass,
> and leveled people from East and West.
>
> Starvation grew,
> as it prowled its way across every measure of Egypt
> and headed for the highlands
> to cut people low
> like crops after a harvest
> reaping.

Awful and extraordinary things came to pass during this plague. Among the things Ibn Abī Ḥajala recorded:

> The plague that occurred in the year 449 (1057) covered the earth, and the Great Plague of 749 (1349) was equal to that one in this regard. Nothing has come to pass like that other than those two!
>
> The plague never entered Mecca except during this time. Many people in Mecca and the neighboring villages died

there, as the multitude of reports say. Birds, wild beasts, gazelles, dogs, and cats, all died during the Great Plague, with buboes under the armpits and other plague symptoms. That year, across all the cities of the earth, no one was safe from the plague, except in the city of the Prophet, Medina. Roughly half of those that belong to the animal world died during this plague. The daily mortality rate in Cairo reached twenty thousand. Some said twenty-five thousand, while still others estimated twenty-seven thousand. . . .[5]

One of the sultan's private merchants, Majd al-Dīn al-Isʿardī, mentioned to me that he was made responsible for Cairo's city gates. He remembered that during the months of Shaʿbān (November) and Ramadan (December), the number of dead reached nine hundred thousand persons or more, and this is apart from those who were not registered. Many enclosures surrounding Cairo became empty and were never inhabited after that. The bottom line is that in comparison to this plague, the totality of all others in the past were a drop of water in a sea or a single point on a circle.[6]

As for Damascus, I was there at the time. I witnessed it in a state of chaos, its walls on the verge of collapse. I saw people's loved ones die, one by one, with buboes, and I saw blood and pustules. The plague dismounted at the stopovers outside the city, and its northerly wind instilled fear in every direction.

In the month of Rabīʿ I (April), people gathered to hear the recitation of al-Bukhārī's *Authentic Hadith.* They read the Chapter of Noah from the Qur'an in the prayer nook of the Companions 3,336 times, in accordance with a vision a man had seen. They called on God to lift the plague, but it only increased.

Then the preacher began to include the prayer for relief from the plague in the qunūt prayer and supplications. The people were overcome with submission, humility, supplication, compassion, penitence, and repentance. The sultan's deputy suspended charging fees for building coffins and anything else related to the dead. This was announced in the streets, so people made their own coffins and prepared them, and the streets were filled with processionals.

> Then people throughout the land were called upon to fast for three days. They did so, and stood for prayer in the city's main mosque, just like during Ramadan. Then they went forth on Friday, the 16th of the month, to the Mosque of al-Qadam,[7] and they implored God to expel the plague. People came from all over, including the protected non-Muslims and children. They filled the streets, most of them beseeching God with their tears. Still, nothing changed except for the worse, and the death count only grew higher.
>
> Then, on the second of the month of Rajab (September), in the afternoon, a windstorm swept past, kicking up dust, first yellow, then red, then black, until it darkened the earth. People sheltered for three hours pleading to God and begging His forgiveness until the storm lifted. They hoped that this marked the end of the plague, but the deaths did not decrease, and the plague dragged on until the end of the year. The number dying reached a thousand people per day inside the city walls. The preacher at the main mosque led the funeral prayer over the bodies of sixty-five at one time. That was a terrible affair, and the cause of great tumult in the main mosque.

Someone whom I trust told me that he was a witness to something like that in the Mosque of ʿAmr ibn al-ʿĀṣ.[8] I read the following in Ṣalāh al-Dīn al-Ṣafadī's *The Reminder*:

> The plague began in the year 449 (1057) in Gaza, in Greater Syria. Then it struck Beirut, then all of Greater Syria. It killed through inhalation of polluted air, and by numerous buboes that erupted around sensitive areas of their body, such as the armpits and the like; by pustules behind their ears; and by the cucumber-like buboes in their groin. Some of them spat blood and fell to their death.

And al-Ṣafadī wrote in an epistle:

> Havoc is its pleasure,
> torment is its work.

I speak of the plague,
and tell
of its ill tidings.
Across the land
it afflicted spirit and flesh.

As this year commenced,
it went into Egypt.
People lost their resolve
and were restless.
Death marched upon the soldiers,
assaulting them, committing atrocities,
trembling
the hearts
of creation.
And inflicting misery
in their breasts.

It showed everyone their place
and left no household unwrapped in gauze.
People were between death and dying,
expecting to pass away,
while passing.
The arrogant
awoke each morning
haunted by the thought of death
standing outside their door.

When the plague entered
a house, every last person fled.
But no sooner had they reached the courtyard
than they were cast into its flames
like kindling.
Desires for worldly gain were riven,
and good acts abounded.
People venerated God,
they implored Him, they cried out to Him,
they acted on the saying of the Prophet:

"At dawn do not await the dusk,
at dusk do not await the dawn."

Yes, there are
merits of the plague,
unlike anything
that exists.

The plague does not distinguish
between a man and his kin,
and the instant that the plague grabs
one beloved by all his family—
it does not allow their grieving eyelids
a wink of sleep.
Rather, without the illness lingering
or spreading through his body,
it demolishes the lines
of his descendants,
knocking down
his family
tree.

Across the umma,
the plague tarried,
striking all creatures and countries,
bringing hardship and sorrow,
anguish and heartbreak.
No one had ever heard or seen
a thing like that—what
plague crosses lands from every direction?
From the land where the sun rises
to the land where the sun sets?

This plague makes
the Plague of ʿAmwās
and the Plague of Ashraf
look like pinpricks.
This plague makes

the Girls' Plague
seem like child's play.

Dear God!
We beseech You:
lift this misery—
break this curse
with your unending Mercy.

I read in the book of the Judge of Tāj al-Dīn al-Subkī in the year 764 (1362):

When the plague cast its shadow
upon all souls
bidding farewell to their grief-struck hearts,
it wandered throughout the lands
and spared neither child nor chattel.
It hounded the quarters where people lived,
even the most praiseworthy of places,
spelling doom.

Hair turned gray
as it raided the land of Egypt.
People were occupied in their own affairs,
distracted
from their religious duties,
and taken with sin.

Terror
then entered Damascus, harrowing and grim,
desires were abandoned,
ambitions discarded,
kingdoms came
crashing down.
As choices narrowed,
the gates of peril widened.

How many deaths were caused by the war it waged!
It did not pause, it did not
hesitate.
Its sharp blade drank the blood of the innocent,
until its thirst was quenched.
In this battle, it laid bare
the brazen rage and malice
it harbored.
Its well-trained arrows slaked the bow's wrath.
No defense could be made against it—
no treatment was any use—
all was Divine decree
and heavenly command.
It cut open
a heart,
and pride and spirit
vanished.
If a bubo erupted on a man, he fell
into his grave.
If he spat blood, he would grieve:
Yesterday,
yesterday is lost.

The price of luxuries collapsed
until they were worth but a grain,
as hagglers wept
that their owner met his end.

Many passed before
their time.
Soon all one could hear of
was death.
If the plague seized a person,
his relatives
soon were taken.
If a man was struck,
he would be gone in a day,

and before
long
his entire people were sickened
with disease.

Help us, O
Lord,
Whom
we fear,
Whom
we heed,
Whose
aid and
Whose
reliance
is sought
in all
circumstances.

I read in the hand of our Shaykh Nāṣir al-Dīn Ibn al-Furāt in his *History* that he once attended Friday prayers in the year 749 (1348) on a platform of the mosque of al-Ḥākim. He saw funeral prayers for the dead, who were lined up in three rows, from the first hall to the door of the repository—and the third row was only a little shorter. He lamented: "Death has become so great, it has emptied the streets." He added, "I went out one evening after dusk in the neighborhood of the two palaces, between the sunset prayer and the evening prayer, and walked from the silk market to the chicken market near the mosque of Aqmar. I saw only a few lit lanterns." He also lamented, "Goods were no longer being sold because of the lack of demand. A single pomegranate would sell for half a dinar, and flour from a measure of wheat reached a florin in value." He added, "Explaining that would take a long time; this only begins to scratch the surface."

In my opinion, the plague was grueling in terms of its length. It began at the start of the year, and it did not cease growing until the month of Rajab (September). It was painful during

Shaʿbān (October) and then Ramadan (November); then it abated during Shawwāl (December), and finally lifted during Dhū al-Qaʿdah (January 1349).

That concludes the depictions of the plague that were passed down to us and inform us of the plagues that occurred during the time of Islam. God is the Controller who brings us to an end with grace, and lifts us up to our radiant resting place.

Last Words

I read at the foot of ʿAbdullāh ibn ʿUmar ibn ʿAlī, from Aḥmad ibn Kashtghadī by way of audition, that Najīb al-Ḥarrānī reported to them that Abū al-Faraj ibn al-Jawzī reported to us by way of audition that Abū Manṣūr al-Qazzāz reported to us that Abū Bakr Aḥmad reported to us that Abū Bakr Aḥmad ibn ʿAlī reported to us that Abū ʿAlī ʿAbd al-Raḥmān ibn Muḥammad ibn Faḍāla said that Abū Bakr Muḥammad ibn ʿAbdullāh ibn Shādhān reported to us, "I heard Abū Jaʿfar al-Tustarī saying:

> Abū Zurʿa came to us as he was nearing death. Abū Ḥātim was with him, as were Muḥammad ibn Muslim and al-Mundhir ibn Shādhān, and a group of religious scholars. They began to recite the "Hadith of Giving Instruction"—"Impart the following instruction to those who are dying among you: 'There is no god but God'"—but they were intimidated by Abū Zurʿa, God grant him mercy, and were too nervous to offer him such a lesson. So they said, "Come, we shall recite the hadith."
>
> Muḥammad ibn Muslim started: "Ḍaḥḥāk ibn Makhlad, from ʿAbd al-Ḥamīd ibn Jaʿfar, from Ṣāliḥ . . ." then he lapsed into silence.
>
> Then Abū Ḥātim said, "Bundār narrated that Abū ʿĀṣim narrated from ʿAbd al-Ḥamīd from Ṣāliḥ . . ." but could not get past it, and everyone else remained silent.
>
> So Abū Zurʿa interjected: "Bundār narrated that Abū ʿĀṣim narrated from ʿAbd al-Ḥamīd from Ṣāliḥ ibn Abī

Gharīb from Kathīr ibn Murra al-Ḥaḍramī from Muʿādh ibn Jabal, who said that God's Messenger said:

'He whose last words are "There is no god but God" enters paradise.'" Then he died.[9]

Abū Muḥammad ibn Abī Ḥātim mentioned a shorter version of this story in his biography of Abū Zurʿa:

> I heard my father say that Abū Zurʿa was dying, internally pierced by the plague, with his brow sweating amid the pangs of death. So I asked Muḥammad ibn Muslim, "What have you memorized on imparting to the dying that 'There is no god but God'?"
>
> He said, "Something narrated from Muʿādh." So Abū Zurʿa lifted his head—and he was in the throes of death—and said, "ʿAbd al-Ḥamīd ibn Jaʿfar narrated it . . . ," and he recited the rest of the hadith. The wailing was deafening in the house among those who were present.[10]

The End of the Book Offering Aid on the Merits of the Plague

The author, Ibn Ḥajar al-ʿAsqalānī—may God have mercy on him, may He protect him with His guardian angel, may He place him in His heavenly abode—said: I finished this work in Jumādā II of the year 833 (March 1430) except for the epilogue, which I added during Shawwāl (June) of that same year.
Then I added a little bit more after that.
All praise is for God Alone.
May God bestow abundant peace
blessings upon our master
Muhammad and
his family.

§

APPENDIX

From Ibn Ḥajar's "Journal of the Plague Years"

Excerpts from Ibn Ḥajar's chronicle *Inbāʾ al-ghumr bi-anbāʾ al-ʿumr* (Tidings of the Abundance in the News of the Ages).[1]

THE PLAGUE OF 819 (1416)

Including the Death of Two of Ibn Ḥajar's Daughters

On the twelfth of Muḥarram (March 12, 1416), the Sun moved to the constellation of Aries. It was the beginning of the spring season. The plague began in Cairo, and by the middle of the month of Ṣafar (April), it was taking a hundred souls a day. By the end of Ṣafar, it had increased to two hundred a day. It continued to multiply in that fashion until most people in any given household had died.

The pestilence increased in Upper Egypt and on the coast, until it could be said that most of the people in the village of Huwwa had been killed. It increased in Tripoli until it was said that ten thousand people had died over the course of ten days.

In Rabīʿ I (May), the number of dead in Cairo reached three hundred a day. By the middle of the month, the number reached five hundred. In reality, the number reached a thousand a day because those counted were just those the government recorded. But there were countless numbers of people whom the government did not record.

Two of my own daughters died—ʿĀliya and Fāṭima. A few of my dependents died as well. Except for a few, everyone who was pierced with the plague died quickly.

The plague spread across the lands until it was reported that only a few people in Isfahan remained. The people of Fez counted the number of the dead in one month, and it reached thirty-six thousand; it was as if the entire country lost its people. The Ustādār was occupied with managing the division of the estates of the dead.*

In Cairo, the number of the dead per day began to decrease in the middle of Rabīʿ I (May). By the first of Rabīʿ II (first of June), it was 120, and by the ninth it was twenty-three per day. But the death toll continued to increase in Damascus. It began there in Rabīʿ I (May), and sixty were dying every day by Rabīʿ II (June). By the end of the month, two hundred were dying every day. It increased again in Jumāda II (August).

It likewise struck Jerusalem and Ṣafad and others nearby, but the plague was lifted there in late Rabīʿ I (May). By the twenty-third of the month (June 20), the daily death toll dropped to eleven people.

THE GREAT EXTINCTION: THE PLAGUE OF 833 (1429–1430)

Including the Death of Ibn Ḥajar's Eldest Daughter

In the month of Dhū al-Qaʿda (August), there appeared to a hajj caravan a star from the direction of the coast rising and getting bigger.[2] Then sparks ascended from the star. When they woke up, the heat had become intense. Many a scholar who was walking died, and many of the caravan's donkeys and camels perished.

The affliction of the plague became widespread along the coast. It was said that in al-Maḥalla† five thousand were taken; in nearby al-Naḥarāriyya, it was nine thousand; in Alexandria, 150 died each day; and other places as well. The numbers must be regarded as extraordinary on account of the fact that the plague struck in the dead of winter. Prior to that, there was

*The Ustādār was one of the senior emirs or officials in the Mamluk Sultanate.

†A village north of Cairo.

an outbreak in Bursa and other cities in Anatolia until the death toll was said to have reached more than one thousand every day. When Rabīʿ II (December 1429) ended, the death toll in Cairo was twelve per day; less than a month later, it was approaching fifty per day. By the first of Jumāda I (January 26, 1430), it reached one hundred per day. So the people were summoned to fast for three consecutive days in repentance, and on the fourth day to go out to the desert.

The private secretary and the Shāfiʿī chief judge went out to the desert with them and gathered many distinguished people as well as the general public, and they wailed and cried and begged to God.* They returned back to the city before noon.

But death only increased among them, doubling what it had been. The death toll in Cairo, in particular, reached three hundred every day, excluding those deaths that the government did not record. And in the Nile and in many lakes, fish and crocodiles were found dead, floating belly-up. Countless gazelles and wolves were likewise found that way in the open countryside.

Something extraordinary that occurred during this time was that a ship headed for Upper Egypt that was boarded by forty people did not make it past al-Maymūn—not even a quarter of the way there—before all aboard had died. A hunting party of eighteen gathered together at a certain place, and fourteen of them died in a single day. The remaining four prepared them for burial, but three of the four died while they were out walking. When the last of them arrived at the burial site, he died.

The death toll in Cairo by the end of Jumāda I (February) had reached eighteen hundred a day.[3]

On the fourth of Jumāda I (January 29), the number of the dead in Cairo alone had reached twelve hundred souls. Death struck the Mamluk soldiers of the sultanate, until more than fifty of them died on one day. The count went all the way up to

*The Kātib al-Sirr (private secretary) was the sultan's closest adviser; the chief judge of the Shāfiʿī school was the leading Muslim jurist on the highest imperial court.

505 per day. All the places of worship registered their dead, and the count reached 1,264 souls.

The death struck to the south in al-Qarāfa until around three thousand had died.* Those who carried the dead, washed them, and prepared their graves became so scarce that people dug one large pit and cast the corpses into it. Many death shrouds were stolen. Stray dogs dug up bodies and ate the corpses' limbs. The caskets arrived in such numbers that I saw them lined up all the way from al-Muʾminā prayer hall to al-Qarāfa gate. They were like white vultures circling carrion. In the streets, it was as if the parade of caskets were a long string of camels tied by the tail, one following the other.

In the middle of Jumādā II (March), the sultan's private secretary invited forty nobles, each with the name Muhammad, and distributed money to them. After the Friday prayers at the Azhar mosque, they recited a few simple portions from the Qur'an. When the afternoon prayer approached, they arose and begged God for help and cried out to him. The people who were with them exclaimed "Allahu Akbar!" After that, the forty Muhammads went up to the roof of the mosque, and they all made the call for the afternoon prayer together. When they finished, a foreigner who had migrated to Cairo from Persia turned to the sultan's private secretary and said: "This will lift the plague!" But the plague only increased in its severity.

The plague did not diminish until the start of Rajab (April).

I read a document handwritten by the Ḥanbalī judge Muḥibb al-Dīn: "It was confirmed for me that a person named ʿAlī al-Ḥarīrī had four boats each containing 120 individuals. All of them died of the plague save one."

When the affliction of the plague worsened, the sultan requested a ruling from the learned scholars on how to respond to the striking of the plague. "Does the religious law commend the collective prayers that implore God to lift the affliction? Or the performing of the qunūt during the daily prayers? What did learned scholars in past times do to diminish the plague?"

They wrote the answers to these questions but diverged in

*Al-Qarāfa is a neighborhood in Cairo known as the City of the Dead.

their opinions. In essence, their answer was that supplications, entreating God with humility, and penance were commended; but prior to performing those acts, they recommended undertaking acts of repentance, removal of oppression, and commanding the right and forbidding the wrong. They did not cite anyone from among the pious ancestors who had done that collectively. Rather, they noted that doing them collectively was more conducive to their prayers being answered.

The judge trained in the Shāfiʿī legal tradition answered that performing the qunūt prayer was acceptable because it was a calamity, and al-Shāfiʿī was explicit that performing the qunūt prayer was permissible during times of calamity. Meanwhile, the Ḥanafī- and the Mālikī-trained judges said that performing the qunūt was impermissible. The Ḥanbalī-trained judge answered that, for the Ḥanbalīs, there are two views attributed to the founder of their school; the scholar who permitted it stipulated that the qunūt may only be performed by the head of state, and it must not be performed on a Friday.

The judges and the learned scholars requested the sultan's presence. The rulings were read aloud, and Muḥibb al-Dīn ibn al-Uqṣurāʾī explained it to him. He replied: "I follow the Companions and the pious ancestors, and I do not deviate from them. Rather, everyone should entreaty God in private."

Then the sultan inquired into the meaning of the phrase "oppression," which they had written in their ruling should be removed. The judges and the learned scholars cited a few vague generalities. The sultan said: "I eliminated the reforms that were instituted since the end of the reign of Sultan al-Ẓāhir Barqūq."

The Shāfiʿī judge specified, "Just this year, the following three unjust practices were instituted as reforms: First, pressuring the spice merchants to sell pepper to the sultan, and if they did not do so, they were forbidden from doing business. Second, pressuring the merchants to dump their mineral salt. Third, barring cane sugar from being cultivated except on the sultan's lands." But nothing of consequence resulted from the sultan's response to that.

Instead, the sultan ordered the judges and the emirs to

command the people to repent, abandon their sins, and increase their acts of obedience and other things like that. It was announced in Cairo that women were forbidden from going out to the grave sites. Swindlers were threatened with hanging and women with drowning, and they refrained from it. At that moment, one of his servants came to him and informed him that his eldest son, Muḥammad, had been pierced with the plague.

One of the judges, Zayn al-Dīn al-Tafahnī, saw Ḥusām al-Dīn Dirʿān, the caretaker of the Shaykhūniyya college, who was one of the ones who died this year from the plague, in a dream. In the dream, al-Tafahnī asked Ḥusām al-Dīn about his status in the hereafter. So Ḥusām al-Dīn replied: "Paradise is wide open to the Muslims!" I myself heard this story from al-Tafahnī. Ḥusām al-Dīn was a very good man, of great benefit to the students at the Shaykhūniyya college from the time he took up his position there. He carried out his service to the college in an excellent way.

Among those who died in this year was Zayn Khāṭūn, my daughter. She was the eldest of my children, born in Rajab of the year 802 (March 1400). She learned how to read and write, and I had her hear hadiths from Shaykh Zayn al-Dīn al-ʿIrāqī and Shaykh Nūr al-Dīn al-Haythamī. She was granted permission to narrate their hadiths by those people of Damascus who had unbroken isnads to the Prophet. She died—while pregnant—of the plague. Thus, two martyrdoms combined in her.

THE PLAGUE OF 848 (1444)

Ibn Ḥajar Is Struck by Plague

Beginning Monday, the first of Muḥarram (April 20), the plague began to gradually increase, until the deaths each day exceeded 120 among those who registered for inheritances. It was said that it exceeded two hundred a day, and most of those who died were slaves and children. It continued to gradually increase and intensified its fire-like spread until it penetrated the pilgrimage, and increased further, and throngs of the pilgrims' slaves and children died. It was said that the death toll may have reached a thousand a day.

On Friday, Ṣafar 3 (May 22), after the Friday prayers, as the sun's state was that of the third month of the solar year, and the skies rained lightly without thunder a tempestuous dust storm, which then subsided. The people began to chatter among themselves that the pestilence had abated after its peak.

On Sunday night, the fifth of Ṣafar (May 24), I discovered a pain under my right armpit and a prickly source of discomfort, but went to sleep despite it. The next day, the pain increased slightly. So I went back to sleep in acceptance and full recognition that the affliction remained unchanged. By the tenth, it appeared under my armpit like a soft plum. After that, it lightened little by little until only a final portion of it remained.

Then it went away as if it had never been—praise be to God.

Glossary and Register of Proper Names

Abū Dāwūd (d. 888). Preeminent hadith collector, whose principal work is ranked by Sunnis to be among the six canonical collections of hadiths. He studied in Baghdad under another giant in the discipline of the hadith sciences, Aḥmad ibn Ḥanbal.

Abū Hurayra (d. ca. 678). Famous Companion to Muhammad. Many thousands of hadiths are traced through him, more than through any other Companion. Known for both piety and humor, Abū Hurayra was briefly appointed governor of Bahrain.

Abū ʿUbayda ibn al-Jarrāḥ (d. 639). Abū ʿUbayda was a member of the Prophet's innermost circle and was considered a candidate, alongside figures like Abū Bakr, ʿUmar, and ʿUthmān, to lead Muslims as caliph after Muhammad's death. Later in life, he commanded troops in Syria and became governor there, where he fell victim to the Plague of ʿAmwās.

Aḥmad ibn Ḥanbal (d. 855). Foundational figure in the disciplines of hadith and law, Aḥmad ibn Ḥanbal—Imām Aḥmad, or just Aḥmad—was the eponym of the Ḥanbalī school of law and was said to have studied nearly eight hundred thousand hadiths in order to collect approximately thirty thousand in his work *Chained Hadith*.

ʿĀʾisha (d. 678). According to Sunni tradition, the Prophet Muhammad's favored wife and daughter of his close Companion Abū Bakr al-Ṣiddīq. One third of the hadiths in al-Bukhārī's renowned hadith collection are traced through her, many of which addressed consequential legal issues. In addition to serving as a major political force during and after Muhammad's lifetime, she also excelled in poetry and medicine.

ʿAmr ibn al-ʿĀṣ (d. 663). A Companion of Muhammad, ʿAmr later helped conquer and govern Egypt during the reign of the caliph ʿUmar. Numerous and notable hadiths are traced through him.

Anas ibn Mālik (d. 712). Anas was Muhammad's servant, a respected Companion, and a prolific hadith transmitter. Hundreds of hadiths are attributed to him; nearly three hundred are included in the revered *Authentic Hadith* of al-Bukhārī and Muslim. Whether or not he lived to be more than a hundred years old is a matter of historical debate.

al-Bukhārī, Muḥammad ibn Ismāʿīl (d. 870). His *Authentic Hadith* is often ranked by Sunnis as "the most authentic book" after the Qur'an. The rigor of his methods for authenticating hadiths was taken to be the highest standard, alongside the collection of Muslim ibn Ḥajjāj.

Companions. For Sunnis, the Companions are a revered generation of Muslims who were associates and friends of Muhammad during his lifetime. The Hadith are transmitted on their authority, and the Companions often feature as important role models themselves.

Ibn ʿAbbās, ʿAbdullāh (d. 688). Muhammad's cousin and Companion, Ibn ʿAbbās was considered a prodigy as a scholar and an influential early interpreter of the Qur'an. Later in life, he became involved in politics; he commanded troops in major battles and governed Baṣra for a period.

Ibn ʿAbd al-Barr (d. 1071). A distinguished hadith scholar from Cordoba, Ibn ʿAbd al-Barr was a judge trained in the Mālikī legal school. He later held a judgeship in Lisbon, where he resided and produced works on hadiths, law, and literature for over two decades.

Ibn Abī Ḥajala (d. 1375). A North African poet and scholar who moved to Cairo and witnessed the Black Death; Ibn Abī Ḥajala recorded an account of the plague, and ultimately succumbed to it himself during a recurrent wave.

Ibn Khuzayma (d. 924). A leading Shāfiʿī jurist and an important hadith scholar from Nishapur who studied with al-Bukhārī and Muslim ibn al-Ḥajjāj. Ibn Khuzayma is known for his prestigious collection *The Authentic Hadith* and his *Book of Unity.* The latter argues for the central role of hadiths in clarifying matters of theology.

Ibn Mājah (d. 887). A leading Sunni hadith collector from Persia, Ibn Mājah is best known for his *Sunan*, which is considered one of the six canonical collections of hadiths most revered by Sunnis; the collection is ranked below the others due to the large fraction of hadiths that contain weaknesses in the isnads.

isnad. The series of names, representing the narrators, found in a hadith that links an utterance or practice of the Prophet Muhammad ultimately to a hadith collector, such as al-Bukhārī (e.g., I heard X cite Y, who cited Z, who heard the Prophet Muhammad say. . . .). Scholars of hadith scrutinize the narrators in an isnad in order to discern whether the hadith is authentic or not.

al-Jaṣṣās, Abū Bakr al-Rāzī (d. 981). Al-Jaṣṣās was an important Ḥanafī scholar from Persia who took up residence in Baghdad, where he was influential among the Ḥanafīs. He is the author of *The Laws of the Qur'an*, which Ibn Ḥajar cites frequently.

Muʿādh ibn Jabal (d. 639). A Companion of Muhammad who took command of the troops in Syria after Abū ʿUbayda fell victim to the Plague of ʿAmwās. Muʿādh was asked to pray to lift the punishment of the plague, but he refused and instead prayed that his family receive "a generous share from this Divine mercy." His family soon died of the plague.

Muslim ibn al-Ḥajjāj (d. 875). Born in Nishapur, Muslim was a foundational figure in the study of hadiths; his *Authentic Hadith* came to be ranked by Sunnis at the top of the six canonical books of hadiths, rivaled only by al-Bukhārī's revered work of a similar stature.

al-Nasāʾī, Abū ʿAbd al-Raḥmān (d. 915). From Khorasan, and later settled in Cairo and then Damascus, al-Nāsāʾī was the compiler of one of the six canonical collections of Sunni hadiths. Ibn Ḥajar ranked his collection just behind the collections of al-Bukhārī and Muslim in terms of the reliability of the hadiths it contained.

Plague of ʿAmwās. This plague raged in Syria between 638 and 640 in the town of ʿAmwās (sometimes spelled ʿAmawās; Latin: Emmaus) near Jerusalem. It was very likely a recurrent wave of the Plague of Justinian, which spread during the sixth century. It features in many important hadiths about the Companions during their conquests there and was a formative moment for the early Muslim community in the decade after the Prophet Muhammad's death.

Qāḍī ʿIyāḍ ibn Mūsā (d. 1149). Born in Ceuta off the coast of Morocco, ʿIyāḍ was a critical figure in the history of Mālikī legal thought and a prominent scholar of the Hadith.

qunūt. A special supplication that may be performed as part of the formal prayer ritual. Depending on one's school, it is performed either immediately before or after the bending down motion of the prayer while the one praying is in a standing position.

al-Shāfiʿī, Muḥammad ibn Idrīs (d. 820). A transformative and foundational figure in the history of Islamic legal theory, al-Shāfiʿī elevated the role of hadiths in the derivation of God's law. He is the eponym of the Shāfiʿī approach to law, to which Ibn Ḥajar adhered.

al-Subkī, Tāj al-Dīn (d. 1369). Born in Egypt, later a Shāfiʿī judge in Damascus, al-Subkī was a master of multiple disciplines and a major influence on the Shāfiʿī legal tradition; he is often cited as an authority by Ibn Ḥajar. He witnessed and recorded a depiction of the grimmest parts of the Black Death in 1349 and died of plague himself several years later.

Successors. The Successors are the pious generation of Muslims after the Companions. While they did not live during the lifetime of Muhammad, many were close with the Companions and helped shape early Islamic society in the Prophet Muhammad's absence. The Hadith is transmitted on their authority.

al-Ṭabarī, Abū Jaʿfar (d. 923). Born in Persia near the Caspian Sea, al-Ṭabarī later settled in Baghdad, where he became a celebrated jurist, historian, and exegete of the Qur'an, and hadith master. His historical and commentarial works were known for their precision, comprehensiveness, and detailed citations.

al-Ṭabarānī, Abū al-Qāsim (d. 971). Born near the Sea of Galilee, al-Ṭabarānī traveled the known Islamic world for decades in search of traditions attributed to Muhammad. He emerged as one of the most consequential hadith collectors of his time, and his hadith collections are often cited by Ibn Ḥajar as sources.

al-Ṭaḥāwī, Aḥmad ibn Muḥammad (d. 933). A major Ḥanafī jurist from Egypt and the author of an important creedal work; but Ibn Ḥajar regularly cites al-Ṭaḥāwī on account of his expertise in hadiths, of which he was also a master.

al-Tirmidhī, Abū ʿIsā (d. 892). Al-Tirmidhī was a foundational master of the hadith sciences and authored one of the six canonical collections of hadiths. He was a student of al-Bukhārī, although his own methods of authenticating hadiths invited much greater scrutiny than that of his teacher.

ʿUmar ibn al-Khaṭṭāb (r. 634–644). Revered by Sunnis, ʿUmar was the second caliph and a major figure who oversaw the greatest expansion of Islamic territory during the conquests. ʿUmar served as an enduring role model for both Muslim political leadership and religious authority, and the significance of his response to the Plague of ʿAmwās should be understood in this regard. He was a close adviser to the Prophet Muhammad; in fact, ʿUmar married his own daughter to the Prophet to solidify the relationship.

umma. This term refers to the entire community of Muslims, encompassing them wherever in the world they may be.

zakat. The alms-tax, one of the pillars of Islam, is an annual payment that must be paid by every Muslim who holds a surfeit of wealth and property beyond their means over the course of a given tax year. The monies are generally to be distributed to the poor and needy, although warriors, zakat collectors, and others can also qualify as recipients.

al-Zamakhsharī, Abū al-Qāsim (d. 1144). A Persian polymath, al-Zamakhsharī was an influential Qur'an commentator, Muʿtazilī theologian, and grammarian.

Notes

PREFACE OF THE AUTHOR

1. Here Ibn Ḥajar describes his table of contents, and details his strategy for noting their isnads (chains of transmission). As we have noted in our own prefatory material, we separated the epilogue (or khatm) from the fifth chapter and added an appendix taken from Ibn Ḥajar's chronicles. We have also modified some of the titles for clarity's sake. As for Ibn Ḥajar's assessments of the authenticity of the isnads, we have preserved representative examples in the footnotes, although some details remain in the prose when they are relevant to the argument. Ibn Ḥajar writes: "I concluded each chapter with a glossary to clarify ambiguous phrases or terms. While, most of the time, I cited hadiths without their isnads, I did, however, give the names of the major collections that recorded them, along with whether they are considered fully credible, of passable credibility, or of weak credibility. Sometimes I was succinct in explaining the cause of their weakness, and at other times I went into detail." See *BM*, 65–70.

CHAPTER ONE: *Origins of the Plague*

1. Ibn Ḥajar provides his own isnad and cites versions from al-Bukhārī, Muslim, and Aḥmad; see *BM*, 73–74.
2. Ibn Ḥajar provides his own isnad; see *BM*, 74.
3. Ibn Ḥajar provides his own isnad and cites the version found in al-Ṭabarānī; see *BM*, 75.
4. Ibn Ḥajar notes differences between different versions of isnads originating in al-Zuhrī; see *BM*, 76.
5. The following, and note 9 in this chapter, offer readers a sense of Ibn Ḥajar's assessment of isnads and comparisons of their variant phrasings: "The same isnad above reaches al-Ṭabarānī, who said, ʿAmr ibn Ḥafṣ al-Sadūsī narrated to us, saying ʿĀṣim

ibn ʿAlī narrated to us, saying, Ibn Abī Dhiʾb narrated to us, citing al-Zuhrī, who cited Sālim (Ibn ʿAbdullāh ibn ʿUmar), who cited ʿAbdullāh ibn ʿĀmir ibn Rabīʿa . . . Muḥammad ibn al-Munkadir, Sālim (Abū Naḍr's client), and ʿAmr ibn Dīnār narrated the hadith above, all of them citing ʿĀmir ibn Saʿd, who cited Usāma. Al-Bukhārī and Muslim record it through this isnad. Some versions have the phrase 'one part of the Israelites were punished by it.' Some versions that al-Bukhārī and Muslim record have the alternative phrase 'one part of the Israelites was punished by it.' In one particular version, 'A man came to Saʿd ibn Abī Waqqāṣ asking him about the plague while Usāma was with him. Usāma responded, "I will tell you. . . ."' This does not contradict the version from Saʿd, the Prophet's Companion. It is possible that its consistency with Usāma's version is due to the fact that he is recounting the hadith Usāma was narrating. Ibn ʿAbd al-Barr was the first to regard the narrations originating in Companions other than Usāma as mistaken. Qāḍī ʿIyāḍ followed his view. But—and God knows best—I do not think it is sound. God willing, we will continue the examination of issues connected to this hadith and a full analysis of its isnad in the fourth chapter." See *BM*, 77.

6. Ibn Ḥajar notes differences in the texts and isnads of this hadith, and considers it sound. He cites the version found in al-Ṭabarānī's *Collection*. See *BM*, 78–79.
7. Ibn Ḥajar provides his own isnad and notes nominal differences between two versions; see *BM*, 81.
8. Ibn Ḥajar cites Ibn Muṭayyan's collection; see *BM*, 82.
9. Ibn Ḥajar: "I found the source of this hadith in the collections of Aḥmad ibn Ḥanbal and al-Nasāʾī (in his large collection) with an isnad whose quality reaches the standards set by Muslim ibn Ḥajjāj. Its isnad contains Thābit al-Banānī, who cited ʿAbd al-Raḥmān ibn Abī Laylā, who cited Ṣuhayb, who cited the Prophet. Ibn Ḥibbān authenticated it. This version does not name David. And it uses the word 'death' instead of 'plague.' At the end, it notes that the Prophet used to say the following after the afternoon prayer: 'God, with Your help I fight and strive.' In a different version, it is after the morning prayer. In another version, instead of 'strive,' he says 'I attack. There is no power nor might except with You.'" See *BM*, 82–83.
10. Qur'an 7:133.
11. Qur'an 7:134.

12. Ibn Ḥajar cites al-Ṭabarī and Ibn Abī Ḥātim's exegeses; see *BM*, 84.
13. Ibn Ḥajar discusses the views of various narrator critics on a pivotal narrator of this hadith named al-Qummī, along with the views of various exegetes on the meaning of the terms "ṭufān" and "rijz"; see *BM*, 84–85.
14. Ibn Ḥajar adds, "Sayyār is a Syrian, and Ibn Ḥibbān records him as one of the trustworthy Successors" and notes that Al-Ṭabarī also records the following relevant story, "from Muḥammad ibn Isḥāq, who cited Sālim Abī Naḍr: 'When Moses settled in the land of the Canaanites, Balaam's people came to him and cried: "This Moses came with the Israelites to expel us from your land."'" See *BM*, 85–86.
15. Qur'an 2:243.

CHAPTER TWO: *Understanding the Plague*

1. Ibn Ḥajar cites al-Ḥarbī's *The Obscurities of the Hadith*; see *BM*, 95.
2. Ibn Ḥajar cites Ibn ʿArabī's commentary on *Sunan al-Tirmidhī*; see *BM*, 95.
3. Ibn Ḥajar cites al-Bājī's *Commentary on the Well-Trodden Path*; see *BM*, 95.
4. Ibn Ḥajar: "Khalīl ibn Aḥmad said the same thing in *The Source*: 'A plague is a pestilence.'" See *BM*, 96.
5. For a more detailed lexical comment from Qaḍī ʿIyāḍ on this matter, see *BM*, 96.
6. Manuscript evidence suggests that al-Nawawī had originally written "elbows" (marāfiq) in lieu of "groin" (marāq), which reflects the state of knowledge on the plague at the time. Ibn Ḥajar and others, after having observed the bubonic plague up close after the peak of the Black Death in the mid-fourteenth century, revised al-Nawawī's phrase to "groin" (marāq), surmising that "elbows" (marāfiq) had been a copyist's error. See Nahyan Fancy and Monica Green, "Plague and the Fall of Baghdad," *Medical History*, 65/2 (2021): 168. We thank Nahyan Fancy for directing us to this anecdote; the translation of al-Nawawī's passage is also informed by Lawrence Conrad, "*Tāʿūn* and *Wabāʾ*: Conceptions of Plague and Pestilence in Early Islam," 297.

7. More detailed remarks from Qaḍī al-Huṣayn and al-Baghawī can be found in *BM*, 98.
8. Ibn Ḥajar: "Al-Bandanījī said that 'the plague blackens a part of the body.'" See *BM*, 98.
9. For the full isnad, see *BM*, 100.
10. Ibn Ḥajar cites al-Bukhārī, Muslim, and Mālik; see *BM*, 102.
11. Ibn Ḥajar cites al-Bukhārī; see *BM*, 102.
12. Ibn Ḥajar cites al-Bukhārī and Muslim; see *BM*, 102.
13. We have omitted a brief lexical discussion here; see *BM*, 103.
14. Ibn Ḥajar cites al-Bukhārī; see *BM*, 104.
15. This is an example of why modern readers might be cautious about concluding that Ibn Ḥajar's belief that the plague was spread by "the pricks of the jinn" was a form of zealous anti-scientism. In fact, Ibn Ḥajar believes that physicians, within the proper boundaries of their discipline, could offer definitive knowledge. See the introduction to this volume for a longer discussion of this issue.
16. Ibn Ḥajar: "Ibn Mājah recorded this hadith from Ibn Masʿūd with a good isnad, and Ibn Ḥibbān and Ḥākim authenticated it, and part of it is cited in Muslim's *Authentic Hadith*." See *BM*, 106.
17. This reflects the state of medicine of the time; when al-Kalābādhī says that the blood is burnt, he means exactly that, because the effect of the excess innate heat ends up burning the humors so that they are not in their natural state. We thank Nahyan Fancy for his assistance on this passage.
18. Qur'an 3:140.
19. Qur'an 4:104.
20. Ibn Ḥajar notes that al-Kalābādhī offers this discussion after citing a report attributed to the Companion ʿAmr ibn al-ʿĀṣ, discussed in the fourth chapter of *Merits of the Plague*.
21. Ibn Ḥajar cites Aḥmad ibn Ḥanbal's isnad; an extended discussion of the isnad is found in *BM*, 109–120.
22. Ibn Ḥajar cites Aḥmad ibn Ḥanbal; see *BM*, 120.
23. The edition we rely on has an extraneous negative particle, the presence of which distorts Ibn Ḥajar's meaning. The original has no such particle. Our translation removes it. For the hadith itself, Ibn Ḥajar cites Muslim; see *BM*, 124.
24. Ibn Ḥajar cites Ibn Mardawiyya's commentary on the Qur'an; see *BM*, 124.
25. Qur'an 6:65.

26. Ibn Ḥajar cites al-Bukhārī and offers a gloss of the Qur'anic verse; see *BM*, 125.
27. We translated this sentence based on a phrasing found in a variant manuscript recorded by Aḥmad al-Kātib; see *BM*, 127n5.
28. Ibn Ḥajar cites al-Qurṭubī's *The Book of Discerning on the Commentary of Muslim* and speculates that the scholar whom al-Qurṭubī left unmentioned is Qāḍī ʿIyāḍ; see a fuller discussion in *BM*, 126–28.
29. The editor of *BM* preserved a nonsensical phrasing here, see *BM*, 128. We have replaced it with what must be the correct phrasing, which is corroborated by MS Madrid, El Escorial, Denenbourg 1510; Casiri MDV, f. 19b.
30. Ibn Ḥajar cites Ibn Abī al-Dunyā, who cited Kardūs al-Thaʿlabī; see *BM*, 128–29.
31. Ibn Ḥajar cites Abū Dāwūd and adds: "In my opinion, the isnad is fair in terms of its authenticity." For a full discussion of the isnad, see *BM*, 129–30.
32. Ibn Ḥajar is a bit ambiguous himself in this passage, but we read him as saying that Ibn Taymiyya rejected universally restricting the meaning of "my community" exclusively to the Companions.
33. Ibn Ḥajar cites Aḥmad ibn Ḥanbal and notes: "the transmitters in the isnad are sound"; see *BM*, 130–31.
34. Ibn Ḥajar cites al-Ḥākim; see *BM*, 131.
35. Ibn Ḥajar cites an isnad from Abū Mālik Saʿd ibn Ṭāriq al-Ashjaʿī, as well as a variant from Aḥmad ibn Ḥanbal, which he describes as conforming "to the high standards of Muslim's *Authentic Hadith*"; see *BM*, 132. A brief line on Arabic pronunciation has been omitted here, as well as more discussion of the isnad.
36. Ibn Ḥajar cites al-Ṭabarānī; see *BM*, 133.
37. Ibn Ḥajar records the full references for the three isnads—omitted here—in *BM*, 134.
38. We have omitted a lengthy discussion of the isnads here and some alternate phrasings; see *BM*, 134–37.
39. The following discussion, which we have omitted from the main text, offers a good illustration of Ibn Ḥajar's research methods. He writes: "I suspected that he relied on Shiblī's book, but that his specification of the narrator that transmitted from Abū Mūsā—as ʿAbdullāh ibn al-Ḥārith—could be an addition on top of the excerpt he took from al-Shiblī. Then I saw in a volume collected by al-Manbijī: 'So says al-Shiblī, but I have searched high and low

in numerous and trusted manuscript copies of Aḥmad's *Chained Hadiths*, and I have only seen the hadith with the wording 'your enemies.' I did not see it in *The Book of Plagues* by Ibn Abī Dunyā, so it seems like al-Shiblī is mistaken on this point.' He added, 'Some of them blame Abū al-Qāsim ʿAbd al-Raḥmān ibn Abī ʿAbdullāh ibn Manda for the mistake—but God knows best.' I would add that Abū ʿUbayd al-Harawī had already mentioned the text with the phrase 'your brother' a long time ago in his *Book of Rare Hadith*. He notes the following in the entry on 'pricking': 'In the hadith, "the pricks of your brothers" refers to a piercing that does not penetrate the body. In some isnads, it is phrased as "the piercings of your enemies," and it is interpreted accordingly.' Abū al-Saʿādāt al-Mubārak ibn al-Athīr adopted al-Harawī's view in his book *The End*, defining 'the pricks of your brothers among the *jinn*' as 'piercings that do not penetrate the body.' It is correct that, as both said, the pricks of the jinn are 'piercings that do not fully penetrate the body.' But as for the phrasing 'your brothers,' I do not know where it can be found in any book of hadiths. I looked in Abū ʿUbayd's *Obscurities of Hadith*, then Ibn Qutayba's book, which is like a commentary on Abū ʿUbayd's book, then al-Khaṭṭābī's book, which is like a commentary on Ibn Qutayba's book, the al-Saraqasṭī's book, which is also like a commentary on Ibn Qutayba's book—I did not find anything in them. Nor did I find anything in al-Zamakhsharī's work. Likewise, I looked in Ibrāhīm al-Ḥarbī's work, which is more comprehensive, better yet, more perfect than all the books above, and I did not find anything in it." See *BM*, 137–38.

40. Ibn Ḥajar: "Abū Dāwūd records this hadith, but with the phrasing 'Every bone upon which the name of God was *not* recited.'" See *BM*, 139.
41. Ibn Ḥajar records some notes by al-Zamakhsharī on spelling and pronunciation in Arabic, omitted here.
42. Qur'an 2:36.
43. Qur'an 18:50.
44. Ibn Ḥajar discusses his sources and research process here; see *BM*, 142.
45. Qur'an 6:108.
46. Qur'an 19:28.
47. Qur'an 45:21.
48. Ibn Ḥajar cites Ibn Mājah and notes, "This hadith's isnad is weak, on account of the weakness of one of its narrators, ʿUfayr ibn Maʿdān." See *BM*, 146.

49. Qur'an 4:40.
50. Ibn Ḥajar cites Abū Saʿīd al-Khudrī, "whose authenticity is agreed upon." See *BM*, 147.
51. This hadith is recorded by al-Tirmidhī, al-Nasāʾī, and al-Ḥākim; see *BM*, 149.
52. Ibn Ḥajar: "The isnad is slightly weak, but it is corroborated by a similar hadith cited by Anas ibn Mālik." See *BM*, 151.
53. Ibn Ḥajar includes an alternate version of this hadith with a weak isnad; see *BM*, 152.
54. Qur'an 3:139 and Qur'an 4:141, respectively.
55. Qur'an 4:76.
56. Ibn Ḥajar cites al-Bukhārī; see *BM*, 156.
57. Ibn Ḥajar cites al-Dārimī, who has recorded "an incomplete but adequate isnad." See *BM*, 156.
58. Ibn Ḥajar cites Anas, adding that "al-Bazzār recorded it, but there it contains a weak narrator in its isnad." See *BM*, 156.
59. Ibn Ḥajar cites Muslim, al-Tirmidhī and al-Nasāʾī; see *BM*, 157.
60. Ibn Ḥajar cites Abū Hurayra and adds an assessment of weaker variants of this hadith with slightly different phrasings recorded by al-Tirmidhī and al-Ṭabarānī. A fuller discussion can be found in *BM*, 157.
61. Ibn Ḥajar cites al-Tirmidhī, "who deemed its isnad to be fairly credible"; he also cites al-Nasāʾī, Ibn Ḥibbān, al-Ḥākim, and al-Ṭabarānī. See full discussion in *BM*, 157.
62. Ibn Ḥajar cites al-Ṭabarānī: "While its narrators are trustworthy, there is a break in the isnad." See *BM*, 158.
63. Ibn Ḥajar cites al-Bukhārī and al-Nasāʾī; see *BM*, 158.
64. Ibn Ḥajar cites al-Tirmidhī: "fairly credibly transmitted by a single isnad." See *BM*, 158.
65. Ibn Ḥajar: "Al-Ṭabarānī recorded it with a decent isnad." See *BM*, 159.
66. Ibn Ḥajar cites Ibn Masʿūd: "Ibn Abī Dunyā recorded it with a decent isnad." See *BM*, 160.
67. *BM*'s version of the text was slightly confusing; we found greater clarity when we consulted the hadith in the actual source that Ibn Ḥajar cites, and we amended our translation accordingly.
68. Qur'an 3:18.
69. In order of their citation: Qur'an 2:163; Qur'an 2:255; Qur'an 3:198–200; Qur'an 3:18; Qur'an 7:54; Qur'an 23:116; Qur'an 72:3; and Qur'an 112, 113, and 114.
70. Qur'an 40:1–3. The hadith is cited in al-Tirmidhī with an anomalous isnad; a fuller discussion can be found in *BM*, 162.

71. Ibn Ḥajar cites Abū Dāwūd and Muslim; see *BM*, 162.
72. Ibn Ḥajar cites al-Bazzār and notes "the transmitters of this hadith are trustworthy"; see *BM*, 162.
73. Qur'an 112, Qur'an 113, and Qur'an 114. Ibn Ḥajar: "According to al-Tirmidhī, the narration contained: 'Recite these chapters three times.'" See *BM*, 162.
74. Ibn Ḥajar: "The isnad is decent." See *BM*, 162.
75. Ibn Ḥajar cites al-Tirmidhī; see *BM*, 163.
76. "Abū Hurayra is said to have cited it; the authenticity of this hadith is agreed upon." See *BM*, 163.
77. Ibn Ḥajar cites al-Tirmidhī; see *BM*, 163.
78. Ibn Ḥajar cites al-Tirmidhī, who "judged it to be authentic." See *BM*, 164.
79. Ibn Ḥajar cites Abū Hurayra; Ibn Abī al-Dunyā recorded it "with an isnad that has some weakness." See *BM*, 164–65.
80. Ibn Ḥajar cites al-Tirmidhī; see *BM*, 166.
81. Ibn Ḥajar cites Abū Dāwūd; see *BM*, 166.
82. Ibn Ḥajar cites Dāwūd; see *BM*, 166.
83. The Arabic uses another name for Satan, "Abū Qitara," which we have translated as "deceitful serpent," a phrase some glossators have used to define "Abū Qitara." Ibn Ḥajar: "Al-Bazzār and Abū Yaʿlā recorded it, and its isnad has Layth ibn Abū Sulaym, who is a weak narrator." See *BM*, 167.
84. Ibn Ḥajar cites al-Ṭabarānī "with a good isnad." See *BM*, 167.
85. Ibn Ḥajar cites Ibn Abī Shayba, al-Ṭabarānī, and al-Bukhārī; see *BM*, 167.
86. Ibn Ḥajar cites al-Nasāʾī, Ibn Khuzayma, and Ibn Ḥibbān; see *BM*, 168.
87. Ibn Ḥajar cites Muslim, al-Tirmidhī, and al-Nasāʾī; see *BM*, 168.
88. Ibn Ḥajar cites Aḥmad ibn Ḥanbal, adding, "The isnad is trustworthy, although I think there is a missing link in it." See *BM*, 168. Omitted here is Ibn Ḥajar's technical discussion of some of the other isnads that are problematic; for a fuller discussion, see *BM*, 169.
89. Ibn Ḥajar cites Abū Dāwūd, al-Nasāʾī, and al-Ḥākim; see *BM*, 169.
90. Ibn Ḥajar cites Ibn Abī Dunyā's *Book of Ecstatic Utterings*; see *BM*, 170.
91. A biography of al-Shāfiʿī written by the famous hadith scholar Ibn al-Ṣalāḥ (d. 643/1245).
92. Qur'an 37:143.

CHAPTER THREE: *Martyrdom and the Plague*

1. Ibn Ḥajar cites al-Bukhārī. See *BM*, 179.
2. Ibn Ḥajar cites similar hadiths transmitted from Abū ʿUbayda and Muʿādh ibn Jabal; see *BM*, 179.
3. In Arabic, al-dummal and al-ḥuzza. See *BM*, 180.
4. Ibn Ḥajar cites Aḥmad ibn Ḥanbal and notes two variant phrasings, one from Aḥmad ibn Ḥanbal and the other from al-Bayhaqī; see *BM*, 179–80.
5. Ibn Ḥajar cites al-Bukhārī; see *BM*, 180.
6. Ibn Ḥajar cites Muslim and two variants from Aḥmad ibn Ḥanbal; see *BM*, 180.
7. Ibn Ḥajar cites Abū Dāwūd al-Ṭayālisī; see *BM*, 180.
8. Ibn Ḥajar cites Ibn Abī Shayba and notes that its isnad is strong; see *BM*, 181.
9. Ibn Ḥajar cites Aḥmad ibn Ḥanbal, Abū Dāwūd, and al-Nasāʾī, and notes that Ibn Ḥibbān and al-Ḥākim authenticated it and that Ibn ʿAbd al-Barr said the isnad was excellent. Ibn Ḥajar cites several other isnads for this hadith that are weaker. See *BM*, 181–82.
10. Ibn Ḥajar: "Aḥmad, al-Bazzār, and al-Ṭabarānī recorded it with isnads, one of which is fair." See *BM*, 182.
11. Ibn Ḥajar cites al-Ṭabarānī; see *BM*, 183.
12. Ibn Ḥajar cites Abū Dāwūd; see *BM*, 183.
13. Ibn Ḥajar cites al-Tirmidhī, as well as al-Bukhārī and al-Nasāʾī with slightly different phrasings; see *BM*, 183–84.
14. Ibn Ḥajar cites al-Ṭabarānī; see *BM*, 184.
15. Ibn Ḥajar cites Ibn Ḥibbān; see *BM*, 184.
16. Ibn Ḥajar cites al-Ṭabarānī, who cites Ibn ʿAbbās; see *BM*, 184.
17. Ibn Ḥajar: "Al-Khaṭīb, in his biography of Dāwūd ibn ʿAlī in his *History of Baghdad*, recorded this hadith of the Prophet, citing Ibn ʿAbbās. There is a minor weakness in the hadith's isnad." See *BM*, 185.
18. Ibn Ḥajar: "Al-Tirmidhī recorded this hadith citing Maʿqil ibn Yasār and described it as having an anomalous but credible isnad. God knows best." See *BM*, 185.
19. Ibn Ḥajar cites Muslim, who cites Anas; see *BM*, 187.
20. Ibn Ḥajar cites al-Nasāʾī, who cites Muʿādh; see *BM*, 187.
21. Ibn Ḥajar cites Aḥmad ibn Ḥanbal and al-Ḥākim, who cites Sahl ibn Ḥanīf; see *BM*, 187.
22. Ibn Ḥajar cites Aḥmad ibn Ḥanbal: "Its isnad is good"; see *BM*, 188.

23. Qur'an 22:58. Ibn Ḥajar cites Ibn al-Mubārak's *Book on Jihad*; see *BM*, 188.
24. According to Ibn Ḥajar, Aḥmad cites Muḥammad ibn Ziyād al-Alhānī for this report. See *BM*, 188.
25. Ibn Ḥajar cites Aḥmad ibn Ḥanbal; see *BM*, 188.
26. Ibn Ḥajar discusses some weaknesses with the transmitters; see *BM*, 189.
27. Ibn Ḥajar: "Al-Tirmidhī deemed the hadith to be sound, but singular in its isnad"; see *BM*, 191.
28. Ibn Ḥajar cites al-Bukhārī; see *BM*, 193.
29. Ibn Ḥajar cites Aḥmad ibn Ḥanbal: "The people in its isnad are trustworthy." Ibn Ḥajar offers additional information supporting the reliability of the hadith in *BM*, 194–95.
30. Ibn Ḥajar cites al-Bazzār: "Its transmitters are trustworthy." See *BM*, 195.
31. Ibn Ḥajar cites Aḥmad ibn Ḥanbal, which was authenticated by Abū Yaʿlā, al-Ṭabarānī, and al-Ḥākim; see *BM*, 195.
32. Ibn Ḥajar cites Muslim, who cites Abū Saʿīd al-Khudrī; see *BM*, 195.
33. Ibn Ḥajar cites Aḥmad ibn Ḥanbal: "Its credibility is fair, and its narrators are trustworthy." For a full discussion of the isnad's reliability, see *BM*, 196–97.
34. Ibn Ḥajar cites Aḥmad ibn Ḥanbal and al-Nasāʾī: "This hadith's credibility is sound." For a full discussion of the isnad's reliability, see *BM*, 197.
35. Ibn Ḥajar cites Aḥmad ibn Ḥanbal and al-Kalābādhī; for a full discussion of the isnad's reliability, see *BM*, 197–98.
36. Ibn Ḥajar cites Aḥmad ibn Ḥanbal, al-Bukhārī, and al-Nasāʾī and discusses slight variants in phrasing; see *BM*, 199.
37. Ibn Ḥajar cites Muslim; see *BM*, 200.
38. For instance, one well-known tradition states that one portion of heavenly reward is awarded for offering funeral prayers, while two portions are awarded for attending the burial. See Muslim's *Authentic Hadith* under the "The Book of Funeral Prayers."
39. Ibn Ḥajar cites Muslim; see *BM*, 202.
40. Ibn Ḥajar cites Abū Dāwūd, al-Tirmidhī, Ibn Ḥibbān, and al-Ḥākim; see *BM*, 203.
41. Ibn Ḥajar cites Abū Yaʿlā; see *BM*, 203.
42. Ibn Ḥajar cites Mālik, al-Bukhārī, and Muslim; see *BM*, 204.
43. Ibn Ḥajar cites al-Bukhārī, who cited Anas; for a full discussion of the citation, see *BM*, 204 and 205.

44. We thank Sibtain Abidi for his assistance in translating this passage.
45. Ibn Ḥajar cites by Abū ʿAsīb; see *BM*, 207.
46. Ibn Ḥajar cites Ibn Mājah and a variant from al-Bayhaqī; see *BM*, 209. Ibn Ḥajar notes that some hadith scholars—Aḥmad ibn Ḥanbal, al-Dāraquṭnī, and al-Nasāʾī—found one of the transmitters, Ibn Abī Mālik, to be weak; Ibn Ḥibbān averred that he was an honest man but would make numerous errors. For a full discussion, see *BM*, 210.
47. Ibn Ḥajar cites Mālik and a weaker version from al-Ṭabarānī; see *BM*, 210–11. Ibn Ḥajar speculates in his own endnotes that this bloodshed could refer to battle or the plague.
48. Ibn Ḥajar cites al-Ṭabarānī; see *BM*, 211.
49. Ibn Ḥajar: "This version is even better than the one above"; he cites al-Ḥākim, who said its authenticity conformed to the highest standards set by Muslim ibn al-Ḥajjāj." See *BM*, 211. In the following paragraphs, omitted here, Ibn Ḥajar notes that he heard this hadith himself from an isnad from a female hadith scholar named Fāṭima ibn al-Munjabī, as well as an elevated isnad from a scholar in the Great Mosque in Mecca named Ibrāhīm ibn Muḥammad ibn Ṣadīq. His point is to establish not only the authenticity of the hadith, but also his own scholarly expertise in this area.
50. Ibn Ḥajar cites al-Ḥākim; see *BM*, 212.
51. Ibn Ḥajar cites Aḥmad and Abū Yaʿlā; see a full discussion of reliability in *BM*, 213.
52. Ibn Ḥajar cites Abū Dāwūd with "a fair isnad"; see *BM*, 213.
53. Ibn Ḥajar cites al-Ṭabarānī: "The transmitters of this hadith are trustworthy." See *BM*, 214.
54. Ibn Ḥajar cites Abū Yaʿlā: "The transmitters of this hadith are trustworthy." See *BM*, 214.
55. Ibn Ḥajar cites Abū Yaʿlā with an "authentic isnad"; see *BM*, 214.
56. Ibn Ḥajar cites Ibn Ḥibbān and Abū Dāwūd; see *BM*, 215.
57. We have used the imperfect English terms "premarital sex" and "extramarital sex," but readers should be aware that concubinage constitutes a lawful form of premarital or extramarital sex, at least for men.
58. Ibn Ḥajar cites Aḥmad ibn Ḥanbal "by an authentic isnad from Umm Salama." See *BM*, 217.
59. Ibn Ḥajar: "Muslim recorded this hadith from ʿĀʾisha"; a variant is found in al-Ṭabarānī; see *BM*, 217.

CHAPTER FOUR: *Against Flight from the Plague*

1. Qur'an 2:243.
2. Ibn Ḥajar notes the textual variations of this report as found in al-Ṭabarī and ʿAbd al-Razzāq's Qur'anic exegeses and notes the following additional details in one of the versions: that they were eight thousand in number and that they fled from fighting. See *BM*, 229.
3. For the full isnad, see *BM*, 230.
4. In addition to citing the full isnad, Ibn Ḥajar notes the following from al-Ṭabarī: "There was a man, Ezekiel son of Buzi, who was nicknamed 'Son of the Old Man,' who addressed the people described in Qur'an 2:243, 'those who fled their homes, fearing death, by the thousands. . . .' Ibn Isḥāq added: 'I heard that they left fearing death because of a plague outbreak, or some other sickness that had struck the people . . . then he told the rest of the story.'" See *BM*, 230.
5. For the full isnad, see *BM*, 230.
6. Compare this account with a similar one on the Valley of the Bones in the Hebrew Bible, Ezekiel 37:1–11. Ibn Ḥajar adds: "The isnad for this story contains Asbāṭ as his informant, who cites al-Suddī, who cites Abū Mālik." And later: "While the isnad for this hadith is acceptable, it lacks a narrator who is a Companion. Abū Mālik's given name is Ghazwān; he was a trustworthy narrator from the generation of the Successors. The name of the person who narrated from him is Ismāʿīl ibn ʿAbd al-Raḥmān al-Suddī, who was a minor Successor, and whose narrations are found in Muslim's collection of hadiths." See *BM*, 230 and 232.
7. For Ibn Ḥajar's analysis of the isnad and his note that in some versions of the report, the resurrected exclaimed: "Glory and praise be to You, our Lord. There is no god but You," see *BM*, 232.
8. For Ibn Ḥajar's comparative analysis of the isnads of this report, see *BM*, 233.
9. For Ibn Ḥajar's observations on the isnad of this report, see *BM*, 233.
10. For Ibn Ḥajar's analysis of the variations of this report and his citation of sources that note that the number resurrected were four thousand or over four thousand, see *BM*, 234.
11. Qur'an 4:164.
12. Qur'an 2:243. For Ibn Ḥajar's full citation of this report, see *BM*, 234.

13. After analyzing the isnads of this report, Ibn Ḥajar concludes: "The isnads above, which give the plague as the cause of their fleeing, are stronger and recorded in better sources." See *BM*, 235.
14. Ibn Ḥajar notes, "al-Ṭabarī and Ibn al-Mundhir recorded the report with an authenticated isnad down to ʿAmr ibn Dīnār." See *BM*, 236.
15. Ibn Ḥajar quotes a source as adding the following observation: "Other sources note that they fled from the plague and other people fenced them in by erecting a wall around them. Their bodies decayed and emitted a rotting stench. To this day, you will find that odor emanating from that particular tribe of Jews." For this and his analysis of the isnad, see *BM*, 236.
16. Ibn Ḥajar notes that various sources record the number of the resurrected as three thousand or more, six thousand, eight thousand, nine thousand, ten thousand, thirty thousand, and thirty-one thousand. See *BM*, 237.
17. Qur'an 2:228.
18. Ibn Ḥajar: "Just as a 'julūs' is a plural of 'jālis' and 'shuhūd' is a plural of 'shāhid.' See *BM*, 238.
19. Qur'an 2:96.
20. Qur'an 33:16, Qur'an 4:78, Qur'an 62:8.
21. For Ibn Ḥajar's full citation, see *BM*, 241.
22. For Ibn Ḥajar's full citation, see *BM*, 241.
23. For Ibn Ḥajar's detailed analysis of the isnads and textual variations of this report, see *BM*, 242–45.
24. For Ibn Ḥajar's analysis of the isnads of this report, see *BM*, 245–46.
25. For the full isnad, see *BM*, 246.
26. Al-Bukhārī and Muslim recorded this as well; for the full isnad and variants, see *BM*, 247.
27. For the full citation, see *BM*, 247.
28. For a digression on variants of ʿAbd al-Raḥmān ibn ʿAwf's hadith, see *BM*, 248.
29. Qur'an 2:243.
30. For a number of other well-known versions of the hadith, see *BM*, 250.
31. For variants, see *BM*, 250.
32. For the full isnad, see *BM*, 250.
33. Ibn Ḥajar: "Al-Bukhārī, Muslim, and al-Nasāʾī cite his version." For an extended digression that compares variants among numerous transmitters and analyzes their differences of phrasing, see *BM*, 251–55.

34. Ibn Ḥajar: "The isnad of this hadith has a gap." For the full isnad, see *BM*, 251.
35. Ibn Ḥajar: "There is a gap in the isnad." For the full isnad, see *BM*, 255.
36. The Arabic grammatical construction contains a double negative (lit., "No slave of God . . . without having Diving Reward the likes of a martyr"). We have altered the construction here so the hadith reads naturally in English. For this hadith, Ibn Ḥajar cites al-Bukhārī and several variants; see *BM*, 255–56.
37. For an analysis of the isnad and its variants, see *BM*, 256–57.
38. For variants of this hadith from Ibn Khuzayma, Ibn ʿAdī, Abū Dāwūd al-Ṭayālisī, and al-Ṭaḥāwī, see *BM*, 258.
39. For variants from Ibn Khuzayma and ʿAbd al-Razzāq, see *BM*, 259.
40. Ibn Ḥajar: "The isnad of this hadith also has a gap." For the full isnad and a variant from al-Ṭabarānī, see *BM*, 259–60.
41. For the full isnad, see *BM*, 260.
42. Ibn Ḥajar: "The hadith's narrators are trustworthy, but there is a gap in the isnad." For the full citation, see *BM*, 261.
43. Ibn Ḥajar: "Al-Kalābādhī . . . cites an unidentified man. . . . I view the first isnad, which Aḥmad cited, to be better, with more trustworthy narrators than this one, on account of the unknown narrator. . . ." For a full comparison of the isnads, see *BM*, 262.
44. Ibn Ḥajar links this hadith to Abū Mūsā's brother Abū Burda and judges it to be more authentic than the hadith attributed to Abū Qilābā. See *BM*, 263.
45. Ibn Ḥajar offers a digression on another hadith that "strengthens Aḥmad's narration on the cause." For more, see *BM*, 263.
46. Ibn Ḥajar cites Abū Yaʿlā; for the full isnad, see *BM*, 263.
47. Ibn Ḥajar offers as examples "the hadiths attributed to Muʿādh and Abū ʿUbayda recorded by al-Kalābādhī." See *BM*, 264.
48. For a full citation, see *BM*, 264.
49. Ibn Ḥajar: "Its isnad has some weakness in it." For a full citation, see *BM*, 264.
50. Ibn Ḥajar: "The hadith's narrators are trustworthy, but there is a gap in its isnad." For the full isnad, see *BM*, 265.
51. For Ibn Ḥajar on the full isnad and two variants, see *BM*, 265.
52. Qur'an 2:147.
53. Ibn Ḥajar: "This isnad is good." For the full isnad and variants, see *BM*, 266–67.

54. Ibn Ḥajar views the transmission of this hadith as containing some problems, including a possible unnamed narrator and confusion over the figures named in the text, as well as other important elements of the phrasing of the text. For more, see *BM*, 268–69.
55. Ibn Ḥajar states that, among others, al-Ṭaḥāwī and Ibn ʿAsākir recorded it as well; for a full citation, see *BM*, 269–70.
56. Ibn Ḥajar cites another version from al-Ṭaḥāwī; for a full citation, see *BM*, 271–72.
57. Ibn Ḥajar: "The phrasing is from Shuʿba's version. The isnad all the way to Abū Mūsā is authentic." For another version, see *BM*, 272.
58. Al-Subkī cites Abū Mūsā al-Ashʿarī, Masrūq, and al-Aswad ibn Hilāl; see *BM*, 274.
59. For the full isnad and a citation, see *BM*, 275.
60. For Ibn Ḥajar's critiques of Ibn Khuzayma's omissions; see *BM*, 275.
61. Qur'an 33:16.
62. Ibn Ḥajar: "Al-Sayāla is a place outside Baṣra. This little story that Ibn ʿAbd al-Barr records is rare." See *BM*, 276.
63. Here we have translated "Miṣr" as Cairo and "al-Fusṭāṭ" as "Old Cairo." See *BM*, 276–77.
64. According to Ibn Ḥajar, Aḥmad ibn Ḥanbal recorded several other versions, as did Ibn Khuzayma and al-Ṭabarānī. For an extended discussion, see *BM*, 277–79.
65. Ibn Ḥajar remarks: "In my opinion, this isnad is weak and has three defects." Ibn Ḥajar references an alternate, well-established version from al-Ṭabarānī, Ibn ʿAdī, Ibn ʿAbd al-Barr, and Ibn Abī al-Dunyā's *The Book of Plagues*. For an extended discussion, see *BM*, 279–80.
66. Ibn Ḥajar provides a full isnad, his own isnad, and alternate versions; see *BM*, 280.
67. In the original Arabic, the servant states, with some ambiguity, "God greets him in the morning at the end of a night's revelry." We have interpreted this in our translation to mean: "He greets them in the morning with *His decree* at the end of a night's revelry" to underline what Ibn Ḥajar understood from this hadith—that the servant was warning his master not to flee from the plague. This interpretation is supported by Ibn Ḥajar's note that follows: "Ibn Abī al-Dunyā . . . mentioned the same story, with the addition, '. . . or death comes as decreed.'" See *BM*, 281.

68. Ibn Ḥajar cites al-Tilmisānī's *Commentary on the Well-Trodden Path*; see *BM*, 281.
69. Ibn Ḥajar addresses the issue of Companions who excessively censured those who fled from the plague in the fifth chapter; see *BM*, 282.
70. For the full isnad, see *BM*, 282.
71. For the full isnad, see *BM*, 284.
72. Ibn Ḥajar cites another version recorded by Ibn Abī Shayba with an acceptable isnad; see *BM*, 285.
73. For a full citation, see *BM*, 285.
74. Ibn Ḥajar is citing from al-Baghawī's *Commentary on the Sunna*; see *BM*, 286.
75. Ibn Ḥajar: "Its isnad is authentic according to al-Bukhārī's criterion." For the full isnad, see *BM*, 287–88.
76. Ibn Ḥajar: "This is something that Abū Mūsā al-Madīnī notes in his book *Addendum to the Anomalies*." See *BM*, 288.
77. Ibn Ḥajar: "The hadith's isnad is authentic." For the full isnad, see *BM*, 288.
78. According to Ibn Ḥajar, al-Bayhaqī's isnad is "acceptable"; for the full isnad, see *BM*, 288.
79. Ibn Ḥajar cites Abū Dāwūd and al-Ḥākim; see *BM*, 291.
80. Concerning what we have translated here as "evil augured from a croaking crow" (ṭīra), we rely on Edward Lane: "The Arabs used to augur evil from the croaking of the crow, and from birds going to the left"; see *AEL*, 1:1904. We follow Justin Stearns in translating ḥāma as "death bird," as a hadith in Abū Dāwūd describes it as "a bird that comes to rest on the grave of a dead man, calling out 'Give me to drink!' until the man is avenged"; see Stearns, *Infectious Ideas: Contagion in Premodern Islamic and Christian Thought in the Western Mediterranean* (Baltimore: Johns Hopkins University Press, 2011), 197n85. For "stomach-serpent" (ṣafar), we follow Lane: "a certain serpent in the belly, which attacks beasts and men, and which, according to the Arabs [of the time of ignorance], passes from one to another more than mange"; see *AEL*, 1:1697. Ibn Ḥajar cites al-Bukhārī; see *BM*, 291.
81. For the full isnad, see *BM*, 291.
82. Ibn Ḥajar adds, "Ibn Khuzayma regarded it as authentic." See *BM*, 292.
83. For a full citation, see *BM*, 293.
84. For an extended discussion of Ibn Khuzayma's use of the hadith, see *BM*, 294–95.

85. For a full citation, see *BM*, 295.
86. For a full citation, see *BM*, 295–96.
87. One issue that Ibn Ḥajar points out is that there may be a missing transmitter; for Ibn Ḥajar's full assessment of the hadith's weakness, see *BM*, 297–98.
88. For additional excerpts from al-Ṭaḥāwī, see *BM*, 299–300.
89. This is excerpted from al-Jaṣṣās's *Laws of the Qur'ān*; see *BM*, 300.
90. Qur'an 33:16.
91. This is excerpted from Ibn al-ʿArabī's *Commentary on al-Tirmidhī*; see *BM*, 304.
92. Al-Zarkashī quotes this in his own volume; see *BM*, 305.
93. Qur'an 2:195.

CHAPTER FIVE: *When the Plague Strikes*

1. Ibn Ḥajar: "Its isnad contains ʿĪsā ibn Maymūn . . . but ʿĪsā is a weak transmitter." See *BM*, 320.
2. Ibn Ḥajar cites a variant recorded by al-Nasāʾī, which al-Ḥākim authenticated; see *BM*, 321.
3. Qur'an 18:28.
4. Ibn Ḥajar: "From the Companion Anas . . . Ibn Ḥibbān and al-Ḥākim authenticated it." See *BM*, 321.
5. Ibn Ḥajar: "From the Companion Salmān . . . al-Tirmidhī recorded it, and Ibn Ḥibbān authenticated the version of it from the Companion Thawbān." See *BM*, 322.
6. Ibn Ḥajar: "Al-Ḥākim authenticated this hadith." See *BM*, 322.
7. Qur'an 59:2.
8. Ibn Ḥajar explains that Millawī made this claim because he was not acquainted with the most authentic version of the hadith on this matter; a fuller discussion can be found in *BM*, 323.
9. Qur'an 11:3.
10. Ibn Ḥajar cites Aḥmad ibn Ḥanbal; see *BM*, 326.
11. Ibn Ḥajar cites al-Ṭabarānī; for a fuller discussion of the isnad and its variants, see *BM*, 326.
12. Ibn Ḥajar cites a variant of the same hadith from Aḥmad ibn Ḥanbal that is "not bad in terms of its attestation in comparison to the previous one." See *BM*, 327.
13. Ibn Ḥajar cites al-Bukhārī and Muslim; see *BM*, 328.
14. Qur'an 44:12.

15. Qur'an 7:23.
16. Qur'an 87:14–15.
17. Qur'an 9:23.
18. Ibn Ḥajar omits other subsidiary matters raised by al-Zarkashī because he did not want to belabor the point; see *BM*, 333.
19. Al-Subkī does not name al-Baghawī, but calls him "the author of *The Refinement*"; likewise, he calls al-Juwaynī simply "al-Imām." We have inserted their names for clarity's sake. Al-Subkī adds that leading Shāfiʿī legal authorities "confirm it as al-Shāfiʿī's view." See *BM*, 335.
20. Ibn Ḥajar adds a technical discussion of how later Shāfiʿīs made sense of this controversy in *BM*, 336.
21. Ibn Ḥajar offers more details on the transmission of this view; see *BM*, 337.
22. This is also a response to the idea that visiting the sick was prophetically sanctioned and encouraged.
23. Qur'an 7:155.
24. Ibn Ḥajar cites al-Ḥākim, who "regards it as authentic." See *BM*, 345.
25. Ibn Ḥajar cites a-Tirmidhī, who "regards it as anomalous. Al-Ḥākim assessed its authenticity and had misgivings about it, as there is weakness in its isnad." See *BM*, 346.
26. Ibn Ḥajar cites Ibn Mājah: "All but one of the narrators are sound, and are cited in the two most authentic collections of hadiths. But there is something potentially suspect in ʿAlāʾ ibn al-Ziyād al-Baṣrī's claim to have heard it from Abū Ḥurayra." See *BM*, 346.
27. Ibn Ḥajar cites al-Tirmidhī and al-Nasāʾī, who give more than one isnad for this hadith, but only "one of which is authentic." See *BM*, 346.
28. Ibn Ḥajar cites Muslim and variant phrasings from Mālik, Abū Dāwūd, and al-Tirmidhī; see *BM*, 346.
29. Ibn Ḥajar cites al-Ṭabarānī; see *BM*, 347.
30. Ibn Ḥajar cites al-Ṭabarānī, al-Tirmidhī, and Ibn Mājah; see *BM*, 347.
31. Ibn Ḥajar cites Muslim; see *BM*, 348.
32. Qur'an 6:82. Ibn Ḥajar: "Abū Nuʿaym records this hadith in his *Book of Knowledge*, with a tenuous isnad." See *BM*, 348.
33. Ibn Ḥajar cites Aḥmad ibn Ḥanbal, who notes that "all of the hadith's narrators are sound"; al-Tirmidhī "regards it as acceptable." Ibn Ḥajar cites a variant phrasing from Ibn Mājah; see *BM*, 349.

34. Ibn Ḥajar cites Ibn Ḥibbān and a variant from Aḥmad ibn Ḥanbal and Abū Dāwūd; see *BM*, 349.
35. For more information on the isnad, see *BM*, 352.
36. Ibn Ḥajar cites al-Tirmidhī, who "deems its isnad to be good," Ibn Ḥibbān, and several other variants; see *BM*, 353–56.
37. Ibn Ḥajar cites al-Bukhārī and Muslim; see *BM*, 356.
38. Ibn Ḥajar cites al-Tirmidhī, who "deemed it adequately authentic"; he cites al-Nasāʾī and Muslim as well. See *BM*, 356.
39. Ibn Ḥajar cites al-Tirmidhī, who "records it with a tenuous isnad." See *BM*, 356.
40. Ibn Ḥajar cites al-Ṭabarānī; see *BM*, 357.
41. Ibn Ḥajar cites al-Bukhārī; see *BM*, 357.

EPILOGUE: *A Record of Plagues*

1. Ibn Ḥajar notes: "We earlier discussed the record for the time of the Plague of ʿAmwās to the plague that occurred in Kufa during the time of Abū Mūsā al-Ashʿarī to the plague that al-Mughīra ibn Shuʿba fled while he was a governor of Kufa, and God decreed that he die of it. That was in the year 50 (670). . . . There was also a plague during the year of ʿAbd al-ʿAzīz ibn Marwān's death in the year 85 (704), although some say 82 (701), others say 84 (703), and others say 86 (705)." See *BM*, 362.
2. Ibn Ḥajar leaves off here without concluding. Later copyists continued to chronicle the plagues in the decades that followed; see *BM*, 370n3.
3. Ibn Ḥajar notes that the recension of the prose-poem was relayed to him by Shaykh Abū al-Yusr Aḥmad ibn ʿAbdullāh ibn al-Ṣāʾigh, whose recension of it was certified by some combination of audition and recitation.
4. Ibn Abī Ḥajala died of the plague in 776/1375. He was a poet from Tlemcen who later settled in Cairo and supervised a Sufi lodge there. For further reading, see s.v., "Ibn Abī Ḥadjala," *EI2* (Robson and Rizzitano).
5. Ibn Ḥajar: "I would add that, according to Ibn Kathīr in his *History*, the number of people who died had a lower bound of eleven thousand and an upper bound of thirty thousand." See *BM*, 380.
6. Concerning the phrase "enclosures" (ḥukūr), this meaning is unique to a dialect in Egypt; Lane, *AEL*, 615–16. Concerning

the phrase "a point on a circle," Lane suggests that an alternate meaning for dā'ir is the wide space of land hemmed in by mountains; see Lane, *AEL*, 1:932.

7. The Mosque of al-Qadam is located in Damascus and holds special significance in relation to the Prophet.
8. The Mosque of ʿAmr ibn al-ʿĀṣ is a famous mosque in Old Cairo.
9. Ibn Ḥajar cites al-Ḥākim, but notes "there is weakness in the isnad." For more, see *BM*, 386.
10. Ibn Ḥajar adds another one of his own esteemed isnads for this hadith, from a variant isnad that also cites Abū ʿĀṣim. He assesses it to be a few degrees of separation from the isnad recorded in Abū Dāwūd that cites Mālik ibn ʿAbd al-Wāḥid citing Abū ʿĀṣim. One might imagine that here Ibn Ḥajar is exemplifying the hadith in preparing his audience to be like Abū Zurʿa in their knowledge of this hadith's isnad. For more, see *BM*, 386.

APPENDIX: *From Ibn Hajar's "Journal of the Plague Years"*

1. We have relied on the passages found at 3:87, 3:437–439, 3:445, and 4:224 in Ibn Ḥajar al-ʿAsqalānī's *Inbāʾ al-ghumr bi-anbāʾ al-ʿumr*, edited by Ḥasan Ḥabashī, 4 vols. (Cairo: Majlis al-Aʿlā li al-Shuʾūn al-Islāmiyya, 1969–1998) for the translation. The dates in these accounts should be taken as approximate rather than precise, as several other historians contemporary to Ibn Ḥajar, such as al-Maqrīzī and Ibn Taghrībīrdī, posit alternate dates for these events. The differences are subtle, sometimes differing by a few days, but at other times Ibn Ḥajar is recorded as having dated an event a month earlier than his other colleagues. More research could discern whether these inconsistences reflect Ibn Ḥajar's intentions, or if they reflect editing errors by him, his copyists, or print editors. However, at the level of seasons and years, Ibn Ḥajar's accounts are consistent with other historians' chronologies of events. Competing accounts of these events in Arabic can be found in Aḥmad ibn ʿAlī al-Maqrīzī, *Al-Sulūk li-maʿrifat duwal al-mulūk*, 8 vols. (Beirut: Dār al-Kutub al-ʿIlmīyya, 1997).
2. The dating here is a bit confusing. Dhū al-Qaʿda (August) is in the summer, not the winter. If this event indeed predated the plague of 833/1429, as Ibn Ḥajar presents it here—implying that

there was a causal chain where the shooting star heralded the coming of the plague—then it should technically have been listed under the year 832/1428, rather than the year 833/1429. However, if it was indeed in 833, then there can be no causal connection between this event and the plague, since it would have postdated it. In that case, it is possible that there was a chronical convention to list meteorological events at the top of each entry, and then follow with news of war and plagues. It is also possible that the shooting star event is misdated, as such mistakes are not uncommon.

3. Al-Maqrīzī identifies this date and the next to be a month later than what is recorded in this edition of Ibn Ḥajar's work. A later date would make more sense here, given that Ibn Ḥajar counts one hundred a day on January 26, 1430; a jump to twelve hundred three days later strains credulity. The chronology is also recorded out of order, which may be another reason to doubt the precision of these dates as they have been recorded here.

Index

Aaron, 10, 11
ʿAbbās, 88–89
Abbasid Dynasty, 193
ʿAbd al-ʿAzīz ibn Marwān, 130, 191, 251n1
ʿAbd al-Barr, 150–51, 233n5, 247n65
ʿAbd al-Ḥamīd ibn Jaʿfar, 217–18
ʿAbd al-Malik, 130, 192
ʿAbd al-Raḥmān ibn ʿAbbās, 59
ʿAbd al-Raḥmān ibn Muʿādh, 121, 122, 134
ʿAbd al-Raḥmān ibn Abī Laylā, 234n9
ʿAbd al-Raḥmān ibn Aslam, 103–4, 105
ʿAbd al-Raḥmān ibn ʿAwf, 5–6, 108, 109–10, 111
ʿAbd al-Raḥmān ibn Ghanam, 115
ʿAbd al-Razzāq, 5, 97, 244n2
ʿAbd ibn Ḥamīd, 97–99
ʿAbdullāh ibn Aḥmad, 47
ʿAbdullāh ibn ʿĀmir ibn Rabīʿa, 233n5
ʿAbdullāh ibn ʿAmr, 61
ʿAbdullāh ibn al-Ḥārith, 36, 237n39
ʿAbdullāh ibn Khubayb, 59
ʿAbdullāh ibn Masʿūd, 62, 122
ʿAbdullāh ibn Saʿīd, 131–32
ʿAbdullāh ibn Thābit, 70
ʿAbdullāh ibn ʿUmar, 63–64
ʿAbdullāh ibn ʿUmar ibn ʿAlī, 217
Abī Mālik, 243n46
Abū al-ʿAbbās al-Qurṭubī, 31
Abū ʿAbdullāh ibn Burayda, 89
Abū ʿAbdullāh al-Manbijī al-Ṣāliḥī al-Ḥanbalī. *See* al-Manbijī
Abū ʿAlī ʿAbd al-Raḥmān ibn Muḥammad ibn Faḍāla, 217
Abū ʿAsīb, 21–22, 41
Abū ʿĀṣim, 217–18, 252n10
Abū al-Asmar al-ʿAbdī, 64
Abū al-Aswad al-Duʾalī, 22
Abū Ayyūb al-Anṣārī, 56
Abū Bakr Aḥmad, 217
Abū Bakr Aḥmad ibn ʿAlī, 217
Abū Bakr ibn al-ʿArabī, 104, 105
Abū Bakr Muḥammad ibn ʿAbdullāh ibn Shādhān, 217
Abū Bakr al-Ṣiddīq, 33, 118, 182
Abū Burda, 246n44
Abū al-Dardāʾ, 183
Abū Dāwūd, 93, 142, 163, 238n40, 248n80, 250n28, 252n10
Abū al-Faḍl ibn al-Ḥusayn, 26
Abū al-Faraj ibn al-Jawzī, 217
Abū Ḥāmid ibn al-Subkī, 172
Abū al-Ḥasan al-Kiyā al-Harrāsī, 139
Abū al-Ḥasan al-Madāʾinī, 129, 191–92
Abū al-Yusr Aḥmad ibn ʿAbdullāh ibn al-Ṣāʾigh, 251n3
Abū Ḥātim, 217
Abū Hurayra, 20–21, 47, 55–56, 81, 90, 91, 133, 141, 142, 182, 184, 186, 227, 239n60, 250n26
Abū ʿInaba al-Khawlānī, 74
Abū Jaʿfar al-Tustarī, 217–18
Abū Mālik al-Ashʿarī, 34, 120, 244n6
Abū Mālik Saʿd ibn Ṭāriq al-Ashjaʿī, 237n35
Abū Manṣūr al-Qazzāz, 217
Abū Mijlaz, 138

Abū Muḥammad ibn Abī Ḥātim, 218
Abū Muḥammad ibn Qutayba, 38
Abū Mūsā, 17, 33, 36, 38, 118, 123, 124, 126, 134, 138, 237n39
  hadiths of, 91
Abū Mūsā al-Ash'arī, 26, 36, 124–26, 128, 251n1
Abū Naḍr, 233n5
Abū Naṣr al-Tammār, 120
Abū Nu'aym, 132, 250n32
Abū al-Qāsim 'Abd al-Raḥmān ibn Abī 'Abdullāh ibn Manda, 237n39
Abū Qilāba, 31, 116–18, 119
Abū Qitara. *See* Satan
Abū Sa'īd, 131–32
Abū Sa'īd al-Khudrī, 59–60, 186
Abū Ṭalḥa, 106–7, 109
Abū al-Tiyāh, 132
Abū 'Ubayda ibn al-Jarrāḥ, 106–109, 117, 120–27, 136–37, 168, 227, 246n47
Abū 'Ubayd al-Qāsim ibn Salām, 59, 148, 237n39
Abū al-Walīd al-Bājī, 16
Abū Wāthila al-Hudhalī, 122
Abū Ya'lā, 56, 69, 84
Abū Zur'a, 217–18, 252n10
Adam, xxiv, xxv
  mercy on, 171
  in Qur'an, 38
  repentance of, 171
  Satan and, 49
'Adī ibn Arṭāt, Plague of, 192
afterlife. *See* heaven; hell; paradise
Aḥmad ibn Ḥanbal (Ahmad), 6, 36–37, 114–17, 130, 167, 176–77, 227, 234n9, 237n35, 237n39, 240n88, 242n29, 242nn33–36, 243n46, 247n64, 249n12, 250n33
Aḥmad ibn Kashtghadī, 217
'Ā'isha, 21, 36, 70, 80–81, 83–84, 87, 93, 113, 128, 130–31, 161, 163–64, 186, 227
'Alā' al-Dīn ibn al-Nafīs, 20
Aleppo, 201–205
Alexandria, xiii, xvii, 220
'Alī ibn Abī Ṭālib, 7–8, 61, 186–87
'Alī ibn Zayd ibn Jad'ān, 129
'Alīm al-Kindī, 167
'Āliya (daughter), 219
Al Jazeera, xvi
alms-tax, of Ramadan, 55–56
'Āmir ibn Sa'd ibn Abī Waqqāṣ, 111–12, 233n5
'Āmir al-Sha'bī, 37
'Amr ibn 'Abasa, 112–13
'Amr ibn al-'Āṣ, 89, 114, 116, 120–23, 227
'Amr ibn Dīnār, 101–2, 112, 233n5, 245n14
'Amwās, Plague of, 35, 86, 122, 123, 229
  in Damascus, 191
  date of and deaths from, 191
  in Kufa, 251n1
Anas ibn Mālik, 6, 21–22, 50, 62, 228
  hadiths of, 43
Anatolia, 221
angels, 58, 98. *See also* Gabriel
  earthquakes by, 94
  forgiveness and, 52
  heaven and, 75
  by Medina, 21
  of mercy, 75
al-Anṣārī, Zakariyyā, xxx
Antichrist
  martyrdom and, 79
  Medina and, 21, 84–85
apple oil, xxviii, 179
Aqmar, 216
aromatics, xiv, 179
As'ad ibn Zurāra, 19
al-Aṣbagh ibn Nubāta, 186–87
Asbāṭ, 244n6
'Āṣim ibn 'Alī, 233n5
Asmā' bint Abū Bakr, 183
al-Aswad ibn Hilāl, 129
'Aṭā' ibn Abī Marwan, 63

Authentic Hadith (al-Bukhārī), 46, 49, 76, 83, 141, 185, 210
Authentic Hadith (Ibn Khuzayma), 48
Authentic Hadith (Muslim), 21, 22, 43, 49, 128, 236n16, 237n35, 242n38
Averroes, xvi
Avicenna, xvi, 18, 19n, 178–79
ʿAwf ibn ʿAfrāʾ, 50
ʿAwf ibn Mālik, 35
Azerbaijan, 194

Badr al-Dīn al-Zarkashī, 32
al-Baghawī, 136, 250n19
Baghdad
  plague in, 193, 194, 195
  siege of, xii
Balaam, xxiv, 9–11, 9n, 92, 235n14
al-Banānī, Thābit, 234n9
al-Bandanījī, 174
Barsbay, Ashraf, xiii, xviii–xix
Baṣra, 193
al-Baṣrī, ʿAlāʾ ibn al-Ziyād, 250n26
al-Baṣrī, Ashʿath ibn Aslam, 100–101
Battle of Nahar, 90, 90n
Battle of Siffin, 90, 90n
Battle of the Camel, 90, 90n
Baybarsiyya college, xviii
al-Bayhaqī, 115, 124–25, 138, 143, 145–46, 243n46
al-Bazzār, 49–50, 120, 131
Bedouins, 38, 58, 140–41, 143
Beirut, 199, 211
The Betrothed (Manzoni), x
al-Bidlīsī, xxxi
Bilāl, 21
birds, 210, 248n80
Black Death. *See* plague
The Black Death in the Middle East (Dols), xxx
bloodletting, xiv, xxviii, xxxivn29, 179
Boccaccio, Giovanni, x
Book of Discerning (al-Qurṭubī), 48–49
The Book of Illness and Expiations (Ibn Abī al-Dunyā), 138
Book of Knowledge (Abū Nuʿaym), 250n32
The Book of Plagues (Ibn Abī al-Dunyā), 237n39, 247n65
Book of Rare Hadith (Abū ʿUbayd ibn al-Qāsim), 237n39
Book of Remembrances (al-Nawawī), 87
The Boundless (al-Zamakhsharī), 37–38
bubonic plague, xxv, 16n, 20n, 176n, 235n6
al-Bukhārī, Muḥammad ibn Ismāʿīl, 5, 21–22, 35, 46, 49, 76, 83, 141, 143, 169, 185, 210, 228, 233n5, 245n33, 246n36
al-Bulqīnī, xviii, 142
Bundār, 217
Burayda, 56–57
Bursa, 221
Byzantine Empire, xi–xii

Cairo
  death rate in, 220, 221
  in Great Plague, 209
  plague in, 172–73, 196, 219, 220, 221
  women in, 223
the Camel, Battle of, 90, 90n
camels, 143–44
camphor, xiv
Camus, Albert, xi
Canaanites, 9–11, 235n14
cane sugar, 223
Casiri, Miguel, xxx
cats, 210
"the cause of death of the righteous before you," 119–26
cautery, xxviii, 19
Chained Hadith (Aḥmad ibn Ḥanbal), 37, 237n39
charity, 171, 172
Christians, xiv, xxv
  jinn and, 41

citrus, xiv
City of the Dead (al-Qarāfa), 222, 222n
civil wars, 35
 battles in, 90, 90n
 jihād before, 166
Collection ('Abd al-Razzāq), 5
Commander of the Believers, 106, 123–26
Commentary on Muslim (Qāḍī 'Iyāḍ), 129
Commentary on Muslim's Authentic Hadith (al-Nawawī), 17
community
 Companions and, 33–34, 237n32
 hadiths on, 28–35
 of Muhammad, 73, 91, 117–18, 164–65
 in paradise, 73, 75, 91
 plague and, 26–36
 praying for, 164–65
Companions, x, 171, 228, 233n5
 community and, 28, 31–32, 33–34, 237n32
 as examples, xxiii
 fighting by, 35–36
 of God's Messenger, 120, 122
 hadiths of, xxiv, 8–9
 jinn and, 37
 on martyrdom, 83
 in Medina, 87
 Muhammad and, 38
 plague and, 113–18
 on plague's cause, 24–25
 praying to God to lift plague, 158
 praying to live longer, 166–67
 in Syria, 110
 'Umar and, 106–7
Concise Book of Medicine ('Alā' al-Dīn ibn al-Nafīs), 20
concubines, xix, 243n57
The Conquests (Sayf), 112–13, 131–32
Conrad, Lawrence, xxxi
contagion, xv, xxv, xxvii, xxxi, 138–48
 mercy and, 180
 al-Qurṭubī on, 180–81
 views on, 181–82
conversion to Islam, 32
COVID-19, xv–xvi
the Cow, 56, 57
Cozbi, 10
crocodiles, 221

Ḍaḥḥāk ibn Makhlad, 217
The Dajjāl. *See* Antichrist
Damascus
 death rate in, 220
 Great Plague in, 168, 210
 Mosque of al-Qadam in, 211, 252n7
 plague in, 169, 191, 195, 196, 199, 214, 220
 Plague of 'Amwās in, 191
al-Dāraquṭnī, 108, 109, 243n46
David, 7–8, 234n9
al-Dāwūdī, 16
Dāwūd ibn 'Alī, 241n17
Day of Judgment, 1
 in Qur'an, 76n
Day of Resurrection, 64, 93
death bird (ḥāma), 248n80
The Decameron (Boccaccio), x
Defoe, Daniel, x
demons
 heavenly rewards and, 48
 Medina and, 85, 86
 Qur'an and, 57–58
 during Ramadan, 46–48
 repelling of, xiv
 safeguards from, 60
The Devil's Traps (Ibn Abī al-Dunyā), 50
al-dhubḥa, 15n, 19
disbelievers
 contagion of, 181
 God's rejection of, 171
 punishment of, 6
The Discerning (al-Qurṭubī), 86, 147–48
The Divine Aid to Victory (*Fatḥ al-Bārī*) (Ibn Ḥajar), xvi, xviii, xx, xxii, 47

dogs, 210, 222
heavenly rewards and, 83
Dols, Michael, xxx

earthquakes, 29, 90, 171
Abū Mūsā on, 91
by angels, 94
heaven and, 6
The Easy Path Forward (Ibn ʿAbd al-Barr), 41
Egypt, xiii–xiv. *See also* Cairo
pestilence in, 219
plague in, 194, 195–97
Eleazar, 11
Encyclopedia (al-Subkī), 174
The End (Abu ʿUbayd al-Qāsim ibn Salām), 237n39
The End (Ibn al-Athīr), 16, 27
The Endpoint (al-Juwaynī), 175
"epidemiological orientalism," xv
The Etiquette of Judges (al-Karābīsī), 160–61
Eve, xxiv
in Qur'an, 38
evil eye, 59–60, 132, 186
Exegesis of the Qur'an (ʿAbd ibn Ḥamīd), 97–99
Exegesis of the Qur'an (ʿAbd al-Razzāq), 97
extramarital sex, 93, 243n57
Ezekiel, xxiv, 98, 99, 100–101, 244n4, 244n6

Faḍāla ibn ʿUbayd, 74
Fakhr al-Dīn al-Rāzī, 42, 104, 105
Farwa ibn Musayk, 141
fasting, xiv
Fatḥ al-Bārī (The Divine Aid to Victory) (Ibn Ḥajar), xvi, xviii, xx, xxii, 47
Fāṭima (daughter of Ibn Ḥajar), xix, 219
Fāṭima ibn al-Munjabī, 243n49
fellowship, 104
Fez, 219–20
fish, 221
forgiveness, 28, 178
angels and, 52
in martyrdom, 44
mercy and, 183, 185
patience and, 184
fornication, xiv
fundamentalism, xv
funeral prayers, 216, 242n38
heavenly rewards for, 83
for martyrdom, 79
at Mosque of al-Qadam, 211
in Mosul, 194

Gabriel, 6, 117
martyrdom and, 86–87
Muhammad and, 61n
on visiting the sick, 186
Galenic tradition, xiv–xv, xxxivn29
The Garden (al-Nawawī), 17
gazelles, 210, 221
Ghāliya (daughter of Ibn Ḥajar), xix
ghazal, xviii, xx
al-Ghazālī, xvi, 18, 110–11, 150
Ghazwān, 244n6
al-Ghifārī, 167
ghudda, 16, 16n
The Gift (Ibn al-Qayyim), 23–24
Girls' Plague, 192
date of and deaths from, 191
Giver of Understanding (al-Qurṭubī), 180–81
God's Messenger (Messenger of God), 36, 37, 112, 182. *See also* Muhammad
on cause of death from plague, 119
Companions of, 120, 122
on contagion, 144, 146
on fleeing plague like march to battle, 130–31
on Gabriel, 86–87
heavenly rewards from, 116
on hell, 46
on martyrdom, 44, 46, 69–70, 72, 74, 77–78, 80, 84–91
on mercy, 183

God's Messenger (*cont.*)
on patience, 184
on praying to live longer, 167
on protection from jinn, 59–62
Qur'an and, 59
Ramadan alms-tax and, 55–56
Satan and, 56–57
on staying in place during plague, 113
on sword, 118
"There is no god but God" from, 218
on the Throne, 58
'Umar and, 106–7, 109, 111
on visiting the sick, 186
"Great Deceiver." *See* Antichrist
The Great Extinction, xiii, xix, 220–24
Great Mosque, in Mecca, 243n49
Great Plague, 195–96
animal deaths in, 210
in Cairo, 209
in Damascus, 168, 210
depictions of, 209–10
in India and Persia, 193
during Ramadan, 210
Greek medicine, xiv
Green, Monica, xii

hadiths, xvi, xxiii
on community, 28–35
contradictions of, xxvii
on divine punishment, 5–6
Ibn Ḥajar and, xvii–xviii, xxii, xxiii–xxiv, xxvii, xxix
on jinn, xxv–xxvi, 26–27, 49–64
on martyrdom, 43–46, 71–73, 77–94
on Medina, xxvii, 19, 22
of Muhammad, xii, 28–29, 241
on plague, 182–87
on plague as divine punishment and mercy, 6
on prohibition from fleeing plague, 99–100
on punishment and mercy, 6
on punishment and upon whom it is sent, 7–12
on staying in place during plague, 113
of "the cause of death of the righteous before you," 119–26
for those who will die, 168–69
on whom is sent punishment of, 7–12
Zayn Khātūn and, xviii
al-Ḥaḍramī, Kathīr ibn Murra, 218
al-Ḥajjāj ibn Yūsuf, 192, 192n
al-Ḥākim, 73, 173, 216, 241n9
al-Ḥalīmī, 47
Ḥamā (city in Syria), 200
ḥāma (death bird), 248n80
Ḥamza al-Zayyāt, 57–58
Ḥanafīs, 117, 177, 223
Ḥanbalīs, 159, 223
al-Harawī, Muḥammad ibn al-Mundhir, 57–58
al-Ḥārith ibn 'Umayra, 120, 121
al-Ḥarrānī, Najīb, 217
al-Ḥasan ibn 'Alī, 186–87
al-Haytham, 125–26
al-Haythamī, Nūr al-Dīn, 224
heaven
angels and, 75
disease sent from, 164
earthquakes and, 6
hell and, 46
seven of, 62
the Throne and, 55n, 57
heavenly rewards
demons and, 48
dogs and, 83
for funeral prayers, 83
from God's Messenger, 116
of martyrdom, x, xxvi, 44–45, 113, 151
Hebrew Bible, xxiv–xxv
Balaam in, 9n
Valley of the Bones in, 244n6
hell, 92
God's Messenger on, 46
heaven and, 46

martyrdom and, 75
Muhammad and, 28
History (Ibn Kathir), 251n5
History (Nāṣir al-Dīn Ibn al-Furāt), 216
History of Baghdad (Al-Khatīb), 241n17
hope, 185
horse, 53–54
Ḥusām al-Dīn Dir'ān, 224

Iblīs, 38, 39n
Ibn 'Abbās, 'Abdullāh, 62–63, 72, 89, 100, 101, 102, 103, 107, 142, 167, 183, 187, 228, 241n17
Ibn 'Abd al-Barr, 16, 41, 127, 129, 153, 228, 241n9
Ibn 'Abdullāh ibn 'Umar, 233n5
Ibn 'Abd al-Malik, Hishām, 192–93
Ibn 'Abd al-Wāḥid, Mālik, 252n10
Ibn Abī Dhi'b, 233n5
Ibn Abī al-Dunyā, 6, 50, 128, 138, 171, 247n67
The Book of Plagues by, 238n39, 247n65
Ibn Abī Ḥajala, 172, 173, 196, 209–11, 228, 251n4
Ibn Abī Ḥātim, 64, 97, 98, 99
Ibn Abī Jamra, 152–53
Ibn 'Adī, 247n65
Ibn al-'Arabī, 15, 151
Ibn 'Asākir, 247n55
Ibn al-Athīr, 16, 237n39
on sword, 27–28
Ibn 'Aṭiyya, 104
Ibn Daqīq al-'Īd, 152
Ibn Ḥajar al-'Asqalānī'. *See specific topics*
Ibn Ḥazm, 41
Ibn Ḥibbān, 235n14, 236n16, 241n9, 243n46
Ibn Isḥāq, 7–8, 117–18, 123
Ibn Jurayj, 112
Ibn Kathīr, 40, 251n4
Ibn Khaldūn, xvi
Ibn al-Khaṭīb, xxxi
Ibn Khātima, xxxi
Ibn Khuzayma, 47–48, 108, 112, 128, 137, 144–45, 146, 153, 228, 247n64
Ibn Mājah, 72, 228, 236n16, 238n48, 243n46, 250n33
Ibn Mālik al-Ashja'ī, 'Awf, 34–35, 90
Ibn Mas'ūd, 37, 55, 82, 144, 150, 236n16
Ibn al-Mulaqqin, xviii
Ibn al-Mundhir, 102, 245n14
Ibn al-Qattān, xvii
Ibn al-Qayyim al-Jawziyya, xxxivn29, 23–24, 51, 94
Ibn Qutayba, 87, 141, 237n39
Ibn Sa'd, 120
Ibn al-Ṣalāḥ, 142, 145–46, 240n91
Ibn al-Sunnī, 161–62
Ibn Taghrībirdī, xix, 252n1
Ibn Taymiyya, xvi, 33–34, 237n32
Ibn 'Umar 'Abdullāh, 36
Ibn al-Wardī, xxviii–xxix, 196
Ibrāhīm al-Ḥarbī, 237n39
Ibrāhīm ibn Muḥammad ibn Ṣadīq, 243n49
Inbā' al-ghumr bi-anbā' al-'umr (Tidings of the Abundance in the News of the Ages) (Ibn Ḥajar), 219–25
India, 193
al-'Irāqī, Zayn al-Dīn, xviii, 224
ISIS, xvi
IslamOnline, xxx
isnads, 229, 234nn6–7
in Abū Dāwūd, 252n10
Aḥmad ibn Ḥanbal on, 36–37, 240n88
of Companions, 26
debates over, 36–37
of al-Ṭabarānī, 233n5
Israelites, 8–11, 111

Jābir ibn 'Abdullāh, 29, 131, 144
Jābir ibn 'Atīk, 82
al-Jābiya, 125, 126

al-Jāḥiẓ, 20
Jaqmāq, xviii–xix
Jaques, Kevin, xxxi–xxxii
al-Jārif, Plague of, 86
Jārif Plague, 191
al-Jaṣṣās, Abū Bakr al-Rāzī, 33, 105–6, 132, 147, 168, 229
Jerusalem, 61, 198, 220
Jesus, xxiv, xxv, 30
Jews, xiv, xxv
  jinn and, 41
jihād, 101, 129
  before civil wars, 166
jinn, xiv
  as "brothers in religion," 93
  as "brothers of humankind," 93
  hadiths on, xxv–xxvi, 26–27, 49–64
  horse and, 53–54
  martyrdom with, 36
  origin of, 38, 39n
  piercing of, 23, 85, 237n39
  possessed by, 49–50
  prick of, 26, 37–43, 46–49, 160, 236n15
  protection from, 54–64, 85
  Qur'an and, 37, 42
  subjugation of humanity by, 51–53
  supplication and, xiv
John the Baptist (Zechariah), 60, 60n
Jonah, 64
Jordan, 125
A Journal of the Plague Year (Defoe), x
al-Juḥfa, 22
Justinian, Plague of, xi–xii
al-Juwaynī, 175

Ka'b al-Aḥbār, 64
al-Kalābādhī, 24–25, 52–53, 80, 117–18, 119, 236, 236n20, 246n47
al-Karābīsī, 160–61
Kātib al-Sirr, 53n, 221n
Kavad II, 191n
al-Kharrūbī, Zakī al-Dīn, xvii
Khaṣṣ Turk, xix
al-Khaṭīb, 241n17
al-Khaṭṭābī, 141, 237n39
Khawla bint Ḥakīm, 63
The Knowledge (Ibn Qutayba), 87
kohl, 49, 49n
Kufa, 251n1

Lane, Edward, 248n80, 251n6
The Laws of the Qur'ān (al-Jaṣṣās), 105–6
Layla bint Maḥmūd ibn Tughān, xx
laylat al-isrā' (the night journey), 61, 61n
leprosy, 17, 19–20, 160
  contagion of, 145
  Muhammad on, 142

Ma'arra, 200
al-Madā'inī, 129–30, 192
maghābin, 19n
al-Maḥalla, 220
Maḥmūdiyya, xix
Majd al-Dīn al-Is'ardī, 210
Mālik ibn Anas, 71, 107, 112, 146, 243n46, 250n28
Mālikīs, 177, 223
al-Malik al-Mu'ayyad, 169–71
Mamluk Empire, x, xiii, xxx, xxxi
  Ustādār in, 220, 220n
al-Manbijī, 33–34, 42, 86, 94, 159–60, 168, 176–77, 237n39
Manzoni, Alessandro, x
Ma'qil ibn Yasār, 241n18
al-Maqrīzī, xix, 252n1, 253n3
martyrdom, xxvi, 151
  categories of, 74–75
  criteria for meriting of, 80–84
  forgiveness in, 44
  funeral prayers for, 79
  Gabriel and, 86–87
  hadiths on, 43–46, 71–73, 77–94
  heavenly rewards of, 113, 151
  hell and, 75
  by intention, 73–75

with jinn, 36
meaning of, 75–76
Medina and, 84–87
mercy and, 69–73, 84–94, 165
al-Millawi on, 162
in paradise, xxvi, 76
of plague, 43–46, 69–94
of plague and battlefield, 79–80
praying for, 77
superior types of, 77–79
of ʿUmar, 168
Mary, 30
Masrūq, 129
Maymūna, 89
The Meaning of the Reports (al-Kalābādhī), 24–25, 52–53
The Meaning of Reports (al-Ṭaḥāwī), 146–47
Mecca, xiii, 87–88
Great Mosque in, 243n49
al-Kharrūbī in, xvii
pilgrimage to, xv–xvi
plague in, 196, 209–10
ʿUmar and, 107
Medicine of the Prophet (Ibn al-Qayyim al-Jawziyya), xxxivn29
Medina, xiii, 134, 136
angels by, 21
Antichrist and, 21, 84–85
demons and, 85, 86
hadiths on, xxvii, 19, 22
martyrdom and, 84–87
ʿUmar and, 107
mercy, 218
on Adam, 171
angels of, 75
contagion and, 180
forgiveness and, 183, 185
martyrdom and, 69–73, 84–94, 165
from Muhammad, 209
of plague, 6
Merits of the Plague. *See specific topics*
Messenger of God. *See* God's Messenger; Muhammad
miasma, xxv
al-Millawī, 86, 161–64
The Mirror (al-Jawzī), 194, 195
Mongols, xii–xiii
Moses, xxiv, xxv, 8, 10–11, 92, 235n14
Mosque of al-Qadam, in Damascus, 211, 252n7
Mosul, 194
Muʿādh ibn Jabal, 56–57, 69, 77, 92, 112–16, 119–22, 159, 166–67, 218, 229
al-Mughīra ibn Shuʿba, 33, 251n1
Muhammad (Prophet), x, xxvi–xxvii
cautery by, 19
community of, 28–29, 33–34, 73, 91, 117–18, 164–65
Companions and, 38
on Companions fighting, 35–36
on contagion, 145, 147
on the Cow, 57
on Day of Judgment, 1
as examples, xxiii
Gabriel and, 61n
on health, 182
hell and, 28
on leprosy, 142
on martyrdom, 70, 71–73, 74, 76, 79, 80
Medina and, 22, 86
mercy from, 209
on patience, 184
on plague's cause, 24–25
on "protection in your countenance," 29
in Ramadan, 49
on Satan and Adam, 49
on staying in place during plague, 113
supplication and, 28, 163–64
on "the sword and the plague," 27–28
in Syria, 112
Muḥammad (son of Ibn Ḥajar), xix
Muḥammad ibn Labīd, 184

Muḥammad ibn al-Munkadir, 233n5
Muḥammad ibn Muslim, 217
Muḥibb al-Dīn, 222
Muḥibb al-Dīn ibn al-Uqṣurāʾī, 223
Mullā Ṣadrā, xvi
al-Mundhirī, 72
al-Mundhir ibn Shādhān, 217
Muslim ibn al-Ḥajjāj (*Authentic Hadith*), 21, 22, 37, 43, 49, 229, 233n5, 236n16, 237n35, 242n38, 243n49, 250n28
Muʿtamir ibn Sulaymān, 185
Muṭarrif ibn ʿAbdullāh ibn al-Shikhkhīr, 132
al-Mutawallī, 17
Muʿtazila, 180
al-Muʾayyad Shaykh, xviii, xxii
al-Muʾminā, 222
myrtle oil, 179

al-Naḍr ibn Shumayl, 75
Nahar, Battle of, 90, 90n
al-Naḥarāriyya, 220
al-Nasāʾī, Abū ʿAbd al-Raḥmān, 56, 59, 229, 234n9, 242n34, 243n46, 245n33, 250n27
Nāṣir al-Dīn Ibn al-Furāt, 216
naturalists, 180
al-Nawawī, 17, 87, 235n6
the night journey (laylat al-isrāʾ), 61, 61n
Noah, xxiv, xxv, 120
  in Qur'an, 210
Notables' Plague, 192

Obedientia et Utilitas, xxx
Obscurities of Hadith (Abū ʿUbayd), 237n39
onions, xiv, xxix, 204
The Origin (Ibn Isḥāq), 7–8
The Ornament (Abū Nuʿaym), 64, 132
Ottoman Empire, xxx, xxxi

paradise. *See also* heaven
  community in, 73, 75, 91
  eighty gates of, 78
  Ḥusām al-Dīn in, 224
  martyrdom in, xxvi, 76
  "There is no god but God" and, xxix, 218
patience, 184
penitence, 210
pepper, 223
Persia, 193
La Peste (Camus), xi
pestilence, 18, 20n
  in Egypt, 219
  plague and, 20–25
  prayers to lift, 161
  repulsion of, 64
Pharaoh, xxiv, 8–9
Phinehas, 11
plague. *See also specific topics*
  in Aleppo, 201–206
  Arabic etymology of term, 15
  bubonic form of, xxv, 16n, 20n, 176n, 235n6
  in Cairo, 172–73, 219, 220, 221
  cause of death from, 119–26
  characteristics and causes of, 15–19
  community and, 26–36
  Companions and, 113–18
  in Damascus, 169, 191, 195–96, 199, 214, 220
  depictions of, 197–217
  as divine punishment, 5–6
  as fleeing from march to battle, 130–31
  hadiths on, 182–87
  heavenly and earthly causes of, 20
  of horse, 53–54
  in Islamic history, xi–xvi
  lawful responses to, 157–74
  as legal life-threatening situation, 174–78
  martyrdom of, 43–46, 69–94
  in Mecca, 209–10
  mercy of, 6
  pestilence and, 20–25
  physicians' advice on protection from, 178–82

pneumatic form of, 176n
praying during calamities, wording of, 173–74
praying to God to lift, 157–66
praying to live longer, 166–73
prohibition of fleeing from, 97–153
protection from, 178–82
staying in place during, 113
in Syria, 115, 192
those permitted to flee, 133–34
in time of Islam, 191–97
ʿUmar's evasion of, 106–11, 126–27
warning for those fleeing, 131–32
who is sent punishment of, 7–12
Plague of ʿAdī ibn Arṭāt, 192
Plague of ʿAmwās, 35, 86, 122, 123, 229
in Damascus, 191
date of and deaths from, 191
in Kufa, 251n1
Plague of al-Jārif, 86
Plague of Justinian, xi–xii
Plague of Salim ibn Qutayba, 192
Plague of Sheroe, 191
poetry, xxviii–xxix
The Positive Laws, 159
premarital sex, 93, 243n57
"pricks of your brothers," 38–43
"pricks of your enemies," 38–43
The Primer (al-Ghazālī), 18
Prophet. *See* Muhammad; God's Messenger
Prostitute's Bridge, 115, 115n, 116

Qāḍī al-Ḥusayn, 175–76
Qāḍī ʿIyāḍ ibn Mūsā, 8, 11, 17, 48, 137, 160, 229
al-Qarāfa (City of the Dead), 222, 222n
Qays ibn Muslim, 124–25
al-Qummī, 235n13
qunūt, 157–74, 157n, 229
Shāfiʿī and, 223
Qur'an, xi, 29
Adam and Eve in, 38
Christian figures in, xxv
the Cow in, 56, 57
Day of Judgment in, 76n
demons and, 57–58
God's Messenger and, 59
on hope, 185
Israelites in, 11
jinn and, xxv, 37, 42
knowledge in, 121
on martyrdom, 43, 76
Noah in, 210
prayer for health and protection from sickness in, 182
Ramadan and, 47
recitations from, xiv
Satan in, 39n
supplication in, 172
thousands in, 103
three periods in, 103
the Throne in, 55–56, 55n, 58, 76
Quraysh, 107, 134
al-Qurṭubī, 48–49, 85–86, 101, 103, 135–36, 147–48, 180–81

Rāba, 122
Ramadan, 48
alms-tax of, 55–56
demons during, 46–48
Great Plague during, 210
Muhammad in, 49
plague during, 197
Qur'an and, 47
The Refinement (al-Baghawi), 250n19
The Reminder (al-Ṣafadī), 211
repentance, 65, 166, 210, 223
of Adam, 171
The Revival (al-Ghazālī), 150
al-rijs, 38
al-rijz, 38
rose oil, xxviii, 179
rubies, xiv
rukūʿ, 157n
The Rulings of the Qur'an (al-Jaṣṣāṣ), 33, 132

Sa'd ibn Abī Waqqāṣ, 70, 233n5
al-Sadūsī, 'Amr ibn Ḥafṣ, 233n5
Ṣafad, 220
al-Ṣafadī, Ṣalāh al-Dīn, 196, 211–14
ṣafar (stomach-serpent), 248n80
Safavids, xxxi
Ṣafiyya bint Ḥuyayy, 49
Sa'īd ibn Jubayr, 8
Sakhbara, 184
al-Ṣalāḥ al-Sulṭān al-Ashraf, 171
ṣalāt, 157n
Ṣāliḥ ibn Abī Gharib, 217–18
Sālim Abī Naḍr, 235n14
Sālim ibn 'Abdullāh ibn 'Umar, 233n5
Salim ibn Qutayba, Plague of, 192
Salmān al-Fārisī, 122, 249n5
salt, 223
Samaritans, 41
Samarqand, 194–95
sandalwood, xiv, 204
sapphires, xiv, 204
sardines, xiv, xxix, 204
Satan, 240n83
  Adam and, 49
  God's Messenger and, 56–57
  in Qur'an, 39n
al-Sayāla, 129
Sayf, 106, 112–13, 131
Sayyār, 9, 235n14
The Sects (Ibn Ḥazm), 41
The Seed of Excellence in Deliverance from the Pestilence (al-Millawī), 161
septicemic plague, 20n
Shaddād ibn Aws, 185
al-Shāfi'ī, Muḥammad ibn Idrīs, 64, 143, 158, 170, 174–75, 230, 240n91
  qunūt and, 223
Shāfi'īs, 158–59, 177, 221, 250nn19–20
  Kātib al-Sirr of, 221n
Shams al-Dīn ibn Khaṭīb Yabrūd, 173
Sharaḥbīl ibn Ḥasana, 69
al-Sharīf Shihāb al-Dīn ibn 'Adnān, 53
Shayba ibn Rabī'a, 21
Shaykhūniyya, xviii, 224
Sheroe, Plague of, 191
al-Shiblī, 38–39, 237n39
Shihāb al-Dīn Aḥmad ibn Yaḥyā ibn Abī Ḥajala, 209
Shīrāz, 193
Shu'ba, 247n57
Shuraḥbīl, 116
Shuraḥbīl ibn Ḥasana, 112–13, 114, 120, 123
Sibṭ ibn al-Jawzī, 194, 195
Siffin, Battle of, 90, 90n
Simeon, 10
Sīs, 205–206
social distancing, xxvii
The Source (al-Shāfi'ī), 158
Source of the Reports (Ibn Qutayba), 38
Stearns, Justin, xxxi, 248n80
stomach-serpent (ṣafar), 248n80
stones, 29
al-Subkī, Tāj al-Dīn, 46–47, 86, 105, 127, 129, 135–36, 139, 140, 165–66, 172, 174, 179–80, 230, 250n19
Sublet, Jacqueline, xxx–xxxi
Successors, 138, 171, 230
  Ghazwān and, 244n6
al-Suddī, 102–3, 244n6
al-Suddī, Ismā'īl ibn 'Abd al-Raḥmān, 244n6
sugar, 223
Ṣuḥayb, 63, 184, 234n9
al-Suhaylī, 37
supplication, xxxiiin10, 117, 172, 210
  abandonment of, 160
  jinn and, xiv
  Muhammad and, 28, 163–64
al-Suyūṭī, xxx
Sweeping Plague, 192
sword, 27–28, 30, 90, 117, 118
Syria, xii–xiii, 211.
  See also Damascus Aleppo; Ḥamā; Sīs; Ma'arra

Muhammad in, 112
plague in, 115, 192, 195
Prostitute's Bridge in, 115, 115n, 116
ʿUmar's evasion of plague to, 105–8

al-Ṭabarānī, Abū al-Qāsim, 5–6, 119, 167, 230, 239nn60–62, 243n46, 247n64, 247n65
isnads of, 233n5
al-Ṭabarī, Abū Jaʿfar, 8, 9, 10–11, 97, 99, 101–2, 103–4, 230, 244n2, 244n4, 245n14
al-Tafahnī, Zayn al-Dīn, 224
al-Ṭaḥāwī, Aḥmad ibn Muḥammad, 106, 133, 134, 135, 146–47, 153, 230, 247n55
Tāj al-Dīn al-Subkī, 214–16
talismans, xiv
Ṭāriq ibn Shihāb, 123, 124–25
ṭaʿūn, 20n
al-Thaʿlabī, 102–3
"there is martyrdom for each," 43–46
"There is no god but God," xxix, 218
thousands, 103
three periods, 103
the Throne, 55–56, 55n, 58, 76
Tidings of the Abundance in the News of the Ages (*Inbāʾ al-ghumr bi-anbāʾ al-ʿumr*) (Ibn Hajar), 219–25
"Tidings of the Plague" (ibn al-Wardī), xxviii–xxix
al-Tirmidhī, Abū ʿIsā, 135, 185–86, 230, 239n60, 239n70, 241n18, 249n5, 250n27, 250n33
Turkistan, 195

ʿUbāda ibn al-Ṣāmit, 70
Ubayy ibn Kaʿb, 56, 58, 173
Ullmann, Manfred, xxx
ulūf, 103–4
ʿUmar ibn al-Khaṭṭāb, 22, 64, 109, 123–25, 230–31
divine will and, 109–10
evasion of plague by, 106–11, 126–27
martyrdom of, 168
return of, 133–34, 136, 137
ʿUmar ibn ʿAbd al-ʿAzīz, 171, 172
Umayyad Dynasty, 192–93
Plague of Justinian in, xi–xii
Umayya ibn Khalaf, 21
umma, 26, 213, 231
Umm ʿAbd, 122
Umm Ayman, 113
Umm Salama, 93
Uns ʿAbd al-Karīm ibn Aḥmad, xviii, xix
ʿUqba ibn ʿĀmir, 58
ʿUraynīs, 135, 140
Usāma ibn Zayd, 5, 8, 111, 112, 233n5
Ustādār, 220, 220n
ʿUtba ibn ʿAbd, 44
ʿUtba ibn Rabīʿa, 21
ʿUthmān, 34
ʿUthmān ibn Abī al-ʿĀṣ, 183
ʿUwaymir Abū Dardāʾ, 122

vaccination, for COVID-19, xvi
Valley of the Bones, 244n6
Varlik, Nükhet, xv, xxxi
vinegar, xiv, xxix, 179
visiting the sick, 186–87

wabāʾ, 20n
The Well-Ordered, 193
The Well-Trodden Path (Mālik), 112
Well-Trodden Paths (al-Dāraquṭnī), 108
wolves, 221
women, xxviii
banned from public spaces, xiv
in Cairo, 223
of Canaanites, 10
The Wonders (al-Harawī), 57–58
World Health Organization, xv

"The Year of Evils," xix
Yemen, xvii, 37, 120, 194
Yersinia pestis, xii, 20n

Zādhān, 167
al-Ẓāhir Barqūq, 223
zakat, 88, 231
al-Zamakhsharī, Abū al-Qāsim, 37–38, 104, 118, 231, 237n39
al-Zarkashī, Badr al-Dīn, 36–37, 39, 135–36, 141, 174, 176, 250n18
Zayn Khāṭūn (daughter), xviii, xx, 224
Zechariah (John the Baptist), 60, 60n
al-Ziftāwī, Tujjār, xvii
Zimri, xxiv, 10–11
Ziyād ibn Abīhi, 192
al-Zubayr, ʿUrwā ibn, 64, 138–39
al-Zubayr ibn al-ʿAwwām, 137
al-Zuhrī, 233n5
Zur, 10

ALSO AVAILABLE

Islam and the Crusades

The Writings of Usama ibn Munqidh

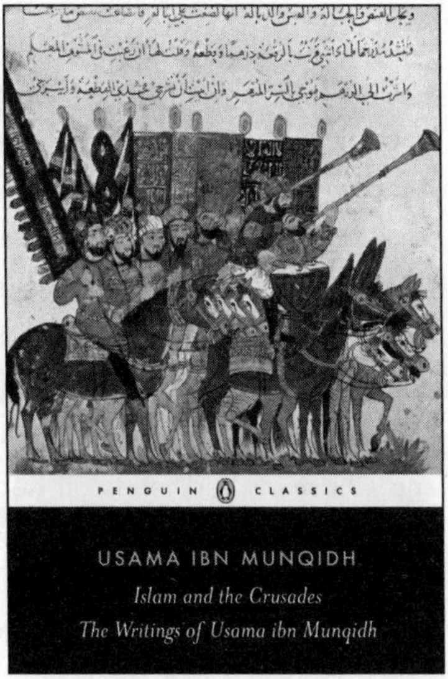

Focusing on Usama ibn Munqidh's *Book of Contemplation* but also including extracts from *Kernels of Refinement* and *The Book of the Staff*, this volume offers a human portrayal of Islamic perspectives on day-to-day existence, warfare, and the curious European invaders. It is a significant contribution to the understanding of the medieval holy wars between Christians and Muslims.

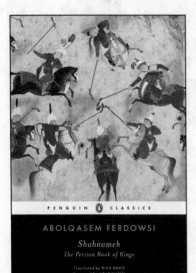

ALSO AVAILABLE

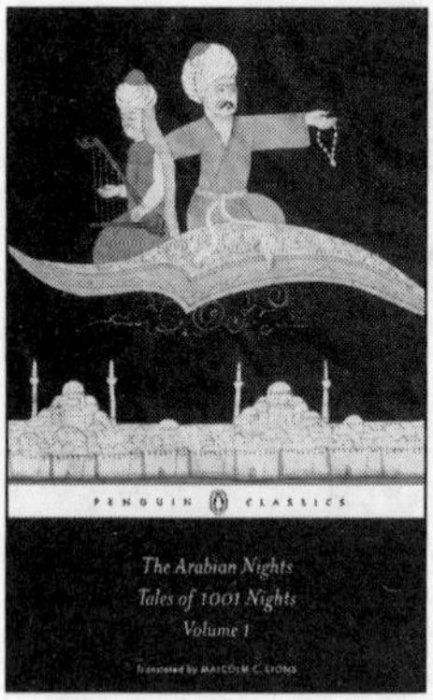

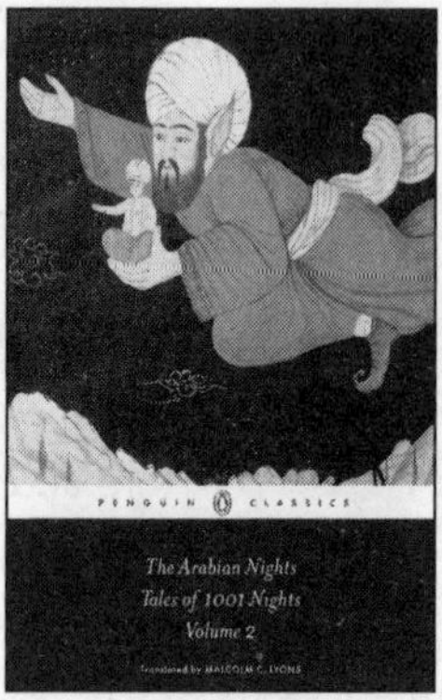

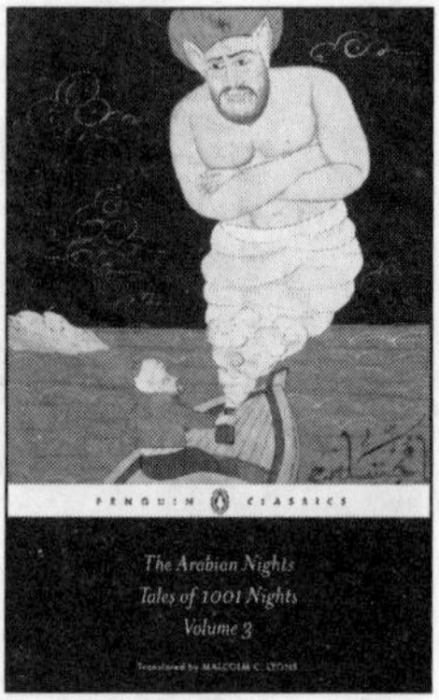

THE ARABIAN NIGHTS: TALES OF 1001 NIGHTS
VOLUMES 1–3

"Magnificent . . . *The Arabian Nights* is not a book to be read in a week. It is an ocean of stories to be dipped into over a lifetime. And this new Penguin edition is the one to have." –*The Sunday Times* (London)

PENGUIN CLASSICS